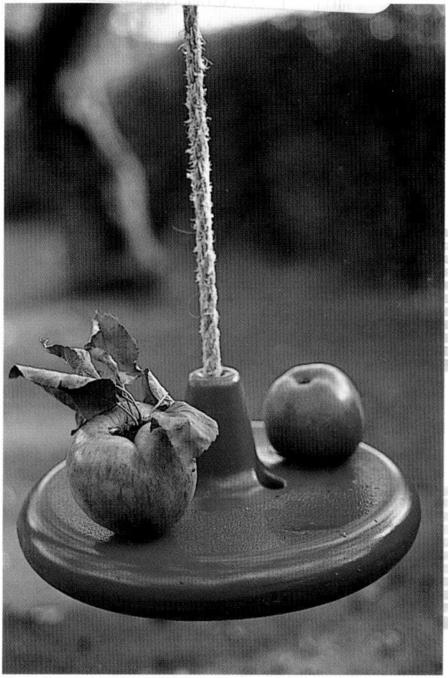

Wonderfoods for kids

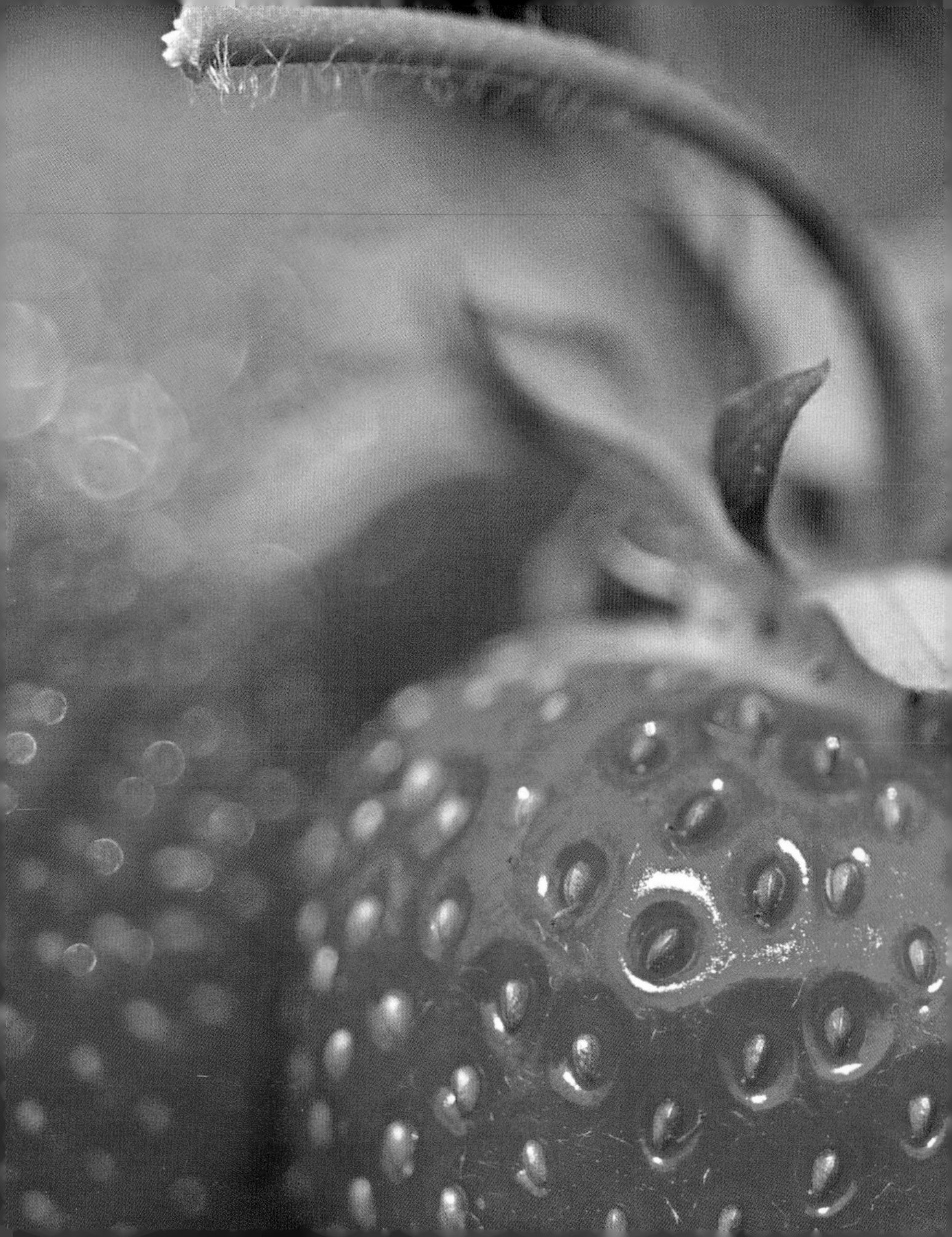

Wonderfoods for kids

Natalie Savona

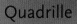

Quadrille

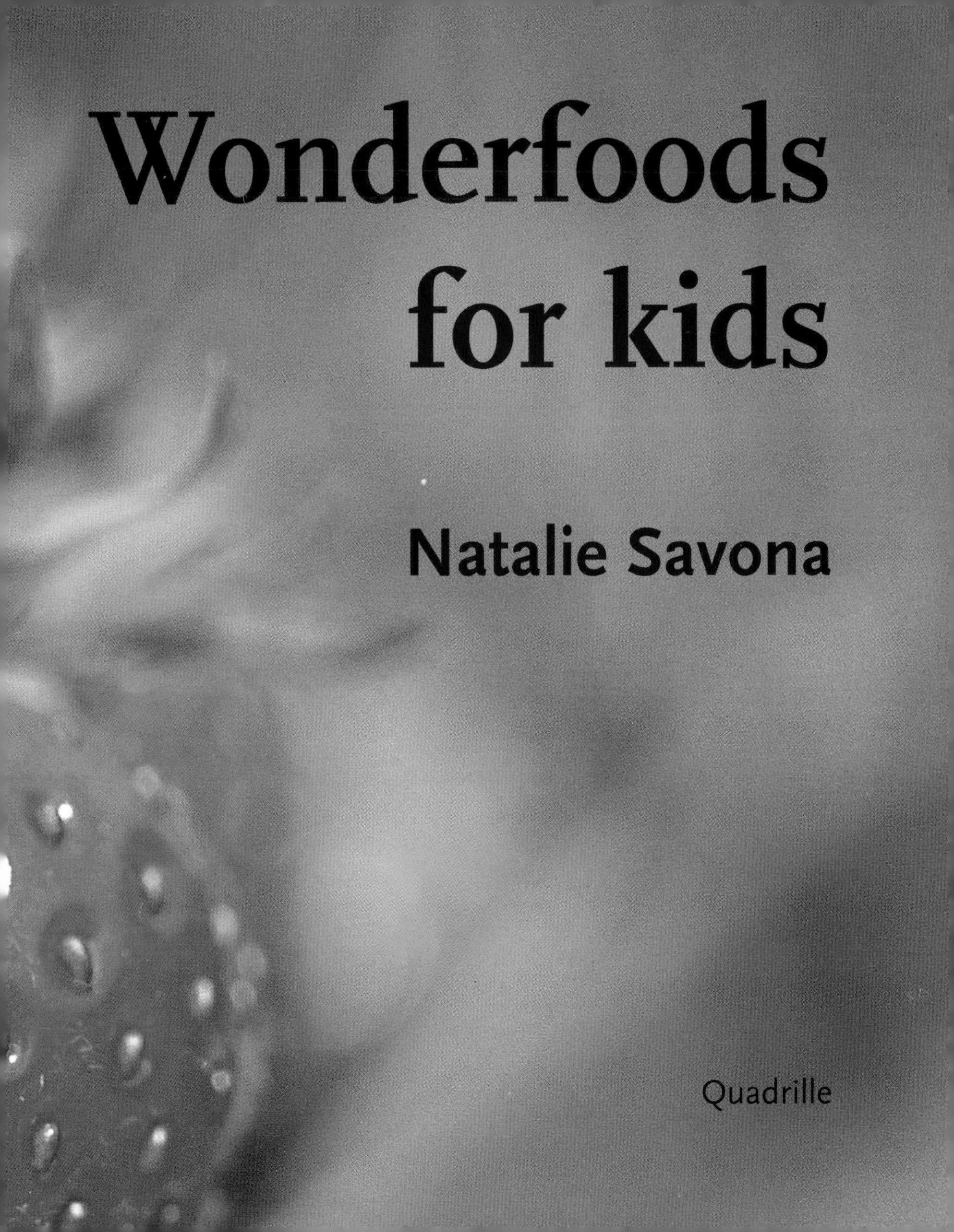

First published in 2006 by
Quadrille Publishing Limited
Alhambra House
27-31 Charing Cross Road
London WC2H 0LS
www.quadrille.co.uk

Cataloguing in Publication Data: a catalogue record for this book is available from the British Library.

ISBN-13: 13: 978 184400 306 8
ISBN-10: 978 184400 306 X

Printed in Singapore

Editorial director Anne Furniss
Creative director Helen Lewis
Project editor Janet Illsley
Designer Ros Holder
Photographer Jill Mead
Production Bridget Fish

notes

Each wonderfood chapter is colour coded, as you'll see from the contents (opposite). However, many wonderfoods benefit several systems or areas of the body. The colour bars alongside the text on each wonderfood highlight other relevant areas.

The number each recipe serves will depend on the ages and appetites of the children and whether you are serving the dish solely to children or to older family members as well. As a rough guide, recipes will serve 4 older children with healthy appetites.

The pink hand symbol denotes recipes that even younger children can help to prepare with supervision.

My measurements are casual, rather than precise. Spoon measures for dry ingredients, like flour, are rounded unless otherwise listed. Liquid measures are obviously level.
1 tsp = 5ml spoon; 1 tbsp = 15ml spoon.
I use a 300ml mug to measure rice, grains etc.

Use fresh herbs, freshly ground black pepper and sea salt unless otherwise stated.

I use medium eggs – organic or at least free-range. I also buy organic poultry.

Timings are for fan-assisted ovens. If using a conventional oven, increase the temperature by 10–15°C (½ Gas mark). Use an oven thermometer to check the temperature.

introduction

Your child already loves wonderfoods – flicking through the book, you'll come across dozens, if not at least some, that appeal. Sure, just like you, there are a few they will screw up their noses at – and some recipes that won't be to their taste. But the foods featured in this book are more than enough for delicious, varied meals that will make for a healthy, happy child with broad food tastes. By basing your child's – and indeed, your entire family's – diet on the foods in this book, you can be sure that he or she will enjoy meals and as an added bonus, will be getting a healthy intake of the full range of essential nutrients. After all, selling a food to a child on the grounds of its health value is never going to be a winner: great taste and fun are.

Simply by focusing your family's food intake on a variety of foods in their natural state, you can barely go wrong. There's nothing mysterious or weird about wonderfoods – as you can see, they're just good, fresh foods that have not been tampered with in factories. Unless your child has a particular allergy, illness or aversion to certain foods, eating a wide selection of these wonderfoods will contribute to his or her well-being, fitness and emotional balance. A few of them are a bit obscure, but these days even large chain supermarkets stock some 'unusual' ingredients (like shiitake mushrooms and quinoa) and what with internet shopping, the world is your oyster, so to speak. Don't be put off by any unfamiliar ingredients, the recipes will give you great ideas on how to prepare them.

As for the categorisation of wonderfoods, you will see that each one comes under a chapter heading linked to an aspect of your child's health. As you can imagine, many wonderfoods fall into several categories, so although each food is allocated to a particular chapter, the coloured tabs on the side of the pages indicate other chapters in which it could sit quite comfortably.

Try and try again... and again and again

'*Bleugch!*' Your child's face responds melodramatically to a new food as though it were an alien's eyeball. But don't despair, researchers have shown that the more children taste a food they haven't had before, the more likely they are to learn to like it. Children are, it seems, predisposed to reject new foods. In other words, it's worth trying out a new food more than once, even if the initial reaction is strongly '*yuk*'. The younger the child is when this is carried out, the better – a child encouraged to be adventurous with foods from an early age is less likely to be a fussy eater.

That said, the less drama over meals the better. Scientists have found that children whose parents struggle with them at mealtimes are more likely to have a difficult relationship with food as they grow up. Indeed, over-concerned parents can actually encourage children to be more fussy. To promote good eating habits, meals need be relaxed and enjoyable.

Walking the talk

Although cajoling your children into eating healthy foods is instinctive and tempting, let's face it, it rarely works. One of the main ways in which children learn their eating habits is by imitation. Studies have shown that mothers who eat more fruit and vegetables foster the same habits in their daughters, without having to pressure them into doing so. Consequently the daughters are also less likely to be picky eaters, are likely to eat more fruits and vegetables, eat fewer fats and sweets, and are less likely to be overweight. So, leading by example appears to have more clout than mealtime mania and bribery...

Why bother?

You know why it is worth feeding your children and yourself on good, fresh food – it takes a hermit these days to be unaware of the impact of diet on health, behaviour and weight. Jamie Oliver managed to bring into the forefront of the nation's psyche the importance of children eating quality foods devoid of excess sugar, salt and fat. What he did – and very well too – was to highlight a serious issue that many people have been harping on about for some time.

Parents and school staff often remark on the improvements in behaviour, health and academic results when children are eating healthy food. It is tough, though, in a world where advertising and large food retailers play on children's gullibility, peer pressure and pester power. Even the most determined parent may yield to pressure, at least once a child is at school.

Producing foods geared specifically to children is a recent notion. For years, all over the world, children have eaten the same food as adults eat. I grew up eating what my parents ate – no shaped chicken pieces in fatty, salty batter, no smiley faced cartons of yoghurt sporting the latest cartoon fad.

I have witnessed children growing up enjoying delicious healthy food, and yes, having the odd pizza and sweets too. I've seen young children avidly tucking into a meal of brown rice, steamed broccoli and stir-fried tofu. The same children enjoy a tomato, fish and alfalfa sandwich for a packed lunch. And even if those children ate a school meal of chips and ketchup, at least their evening meal was good. It's about doing the best you can, and from as young an age as you can. After all, quoting studies that indicate children fed lots of chips before the age of five are more likely to develop cancer isn't useful.

There's no need to give children the so-called health options of everyday foods, such as low-fat milk and added-fibre cereals. Just giving them foods in their natural states will take care of their growth and energy needs – they do, after all, have higher calorie requirements than adults, weight for weight.

The quality and range of the food that your child eats is one of the most important contributing factors to his or her growth, mental development, energy and ability to fight off illness. Yet in this speedy world where children are vulnerable targets of marketing campaigns for the foods that are least helpful, feeding them has unnecessarily become a minefield.

Preparing wonderfoods

You may cast your eye over some of the recipes in this book and assume they are too sophisticated for your children, but I ask you to give them a go. Be flexible – you can omit or substitute ingredients you're sure will be spat out. And be brave – let your children be the judge of whether they will like something or not.

Think of it this way: a child fed pizzas, crisps, fizzy drinks, sweetened yoghurts, frozen 'fish' pieces or indeed, most of the foods marketed to children is going to be startled by fresh, natural foods that aren't crammed with sugar, salt or other additives. Natural foods are not, initially, going to be particularly palatable to taste buds accustomed to bombardment with flavours other than the actual foods themselves. They are not necessarily going to be that palatable to such a child's mind either. That is not to say that children, like adults, cannot adapt. This wonderfoods book doesn't just contain imaginative recipes but simple, inventive ways of presenting foods to make them more appealing.

Even the recipes with longer lists of ingredients are usually made up of things you can keep in the storecupboard, fridge and freezer. And they rarely call for more than one pan or oven dish. Flick through the book and see the lists of ingredients – keep your cupboards stocked with some of the basics: brown rice, oats and other grains, nuts and seeds, cans of tomatoes, chickpeas, beans and coconut milk, olive oil, tamari, stock powder, Chinese five spice powder, ground cinnamon, sesame oil and honey. Other cooking essentials are fresh lemons, ginger, garlic, onions and miso paste. And keep a good selection of fish, chicken and meat, as well as spinach and peas in the freezer. Then with the simple addition of fresh vegetables and fruit, you can concoct great meals.

You'll see that several recipes use tamari, a type of wheat-free soy sauce that's very salty. Adjust this to your taste, bearing in mind it is still salt. And use spices such as cumin and fresh herbs like mint and basil to flavour foods. Dip into this book for ideas, inspiration and of course the detailed recipes, adapting them to suit your children's tastes. I find it's worth making the time to cook 'properly' most nights. And, of course, you can always make extra to save having to cook the following night.

Cooking with children

Most of us have childhood memories of making something in the kitchen. There's no doubt that children like eating what they have made and it gives them a sense of achievement. If you get children involved in helping with some of the everyday cooking – even just a little stir or threading things on skewers – they are more likely to be interested in and enjoy the results. Time 'lost', because they take longer to do something than you, may well be gained by them gobbling up their meal enthusiastically.

After all, enthusiasm for food, for one of the most basic, essential forms of nourishment is surely equal to an enthusiasm for life, for taking care of oneself and for enjoying one of life's great pleasures.

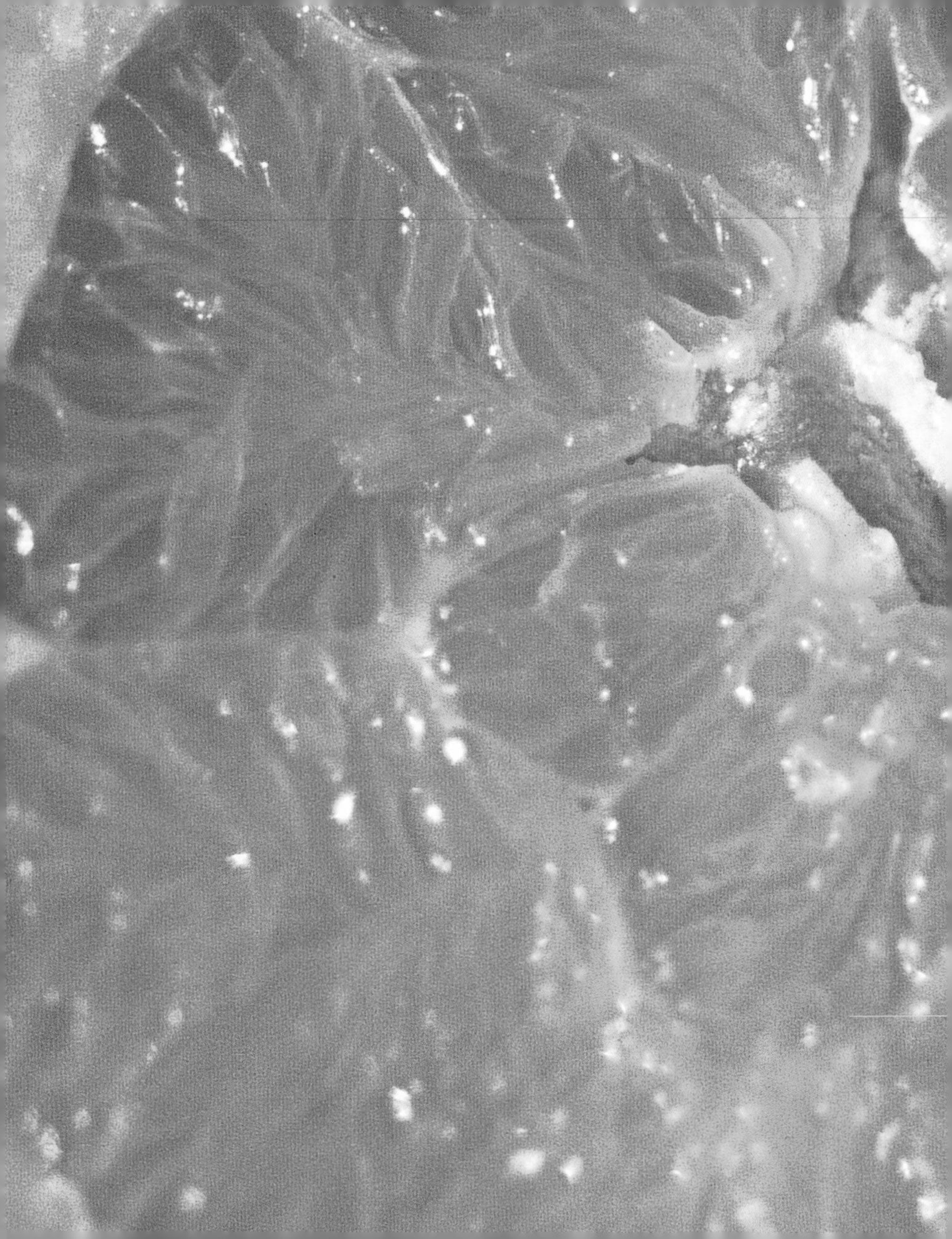

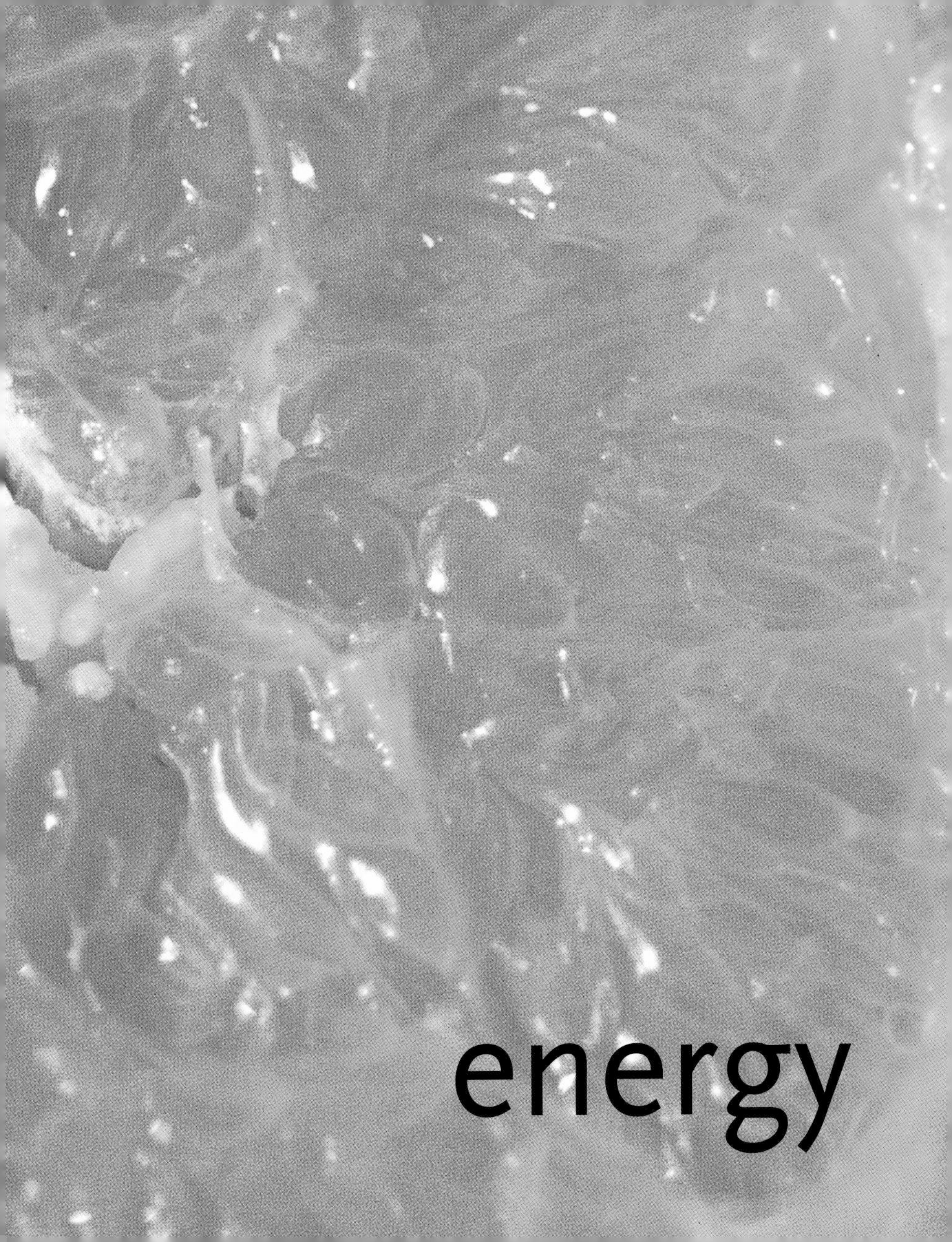

energy

It is generally given that children have boundless energy – sometimes more than parents wish to cope with – but more and more children are tired and listless, or bounding with energy one minute and crashingly tired the next. Fuelling their bodies for good, constant energy is not a simple equation, as most adults know themselves.

Many factors contribute to children's energy levels, for example, the amount of sleep they're getting, how active they are, illness, pressures at school, emotional troubles and many more. Anaemia is a condition that can lead to lethargy, and one that is more likely in a vegetarian or vegan child if care is not taken with their diet. It's important to consider these various factors if your child is lethargic, but the other major issue in your child's energy is, of course, the food that he or she eats. The wonderfoods in this section are loaded with energy. That said, they should form just part of a much wider diet in order to optimise your child's energy.

Most of the energy humans derive from their foods is in the form of carbohydrates, i.e. starchy and sweet foods. These carbs are digested down into blocks of fuel, primarily glucose, which the body can use to actually make energy in each cell. The wonderfoods here are all excellent sources of easily available carbs. Having a regular intakc of carbohydrates, and food in general (e.g. making sure children eat breakfast), is essential for a relatively constant stream of vitality. Children do, however, quickly learn that certain foods give them that feel-good factor relatively quickly. Reliance on such foods is probably the most common dietary pitfall amongst children these days. Foods like sugary breakfast cereals, biscuits and sweets give them a fast energy fix but, just as quickly, leave them crashing. Such speedy fixes are ultimately energy drainers and should only be eaten occasionally. Children who regularly rely on foods of this sort are not only all over the place with their energy levels, but also their mood, concentration and appetite.

On the other hand, a varied diet, which includes foods that give your children energy alongside other important nutrients, such as protein, fats, vitamins and minerals, plus fibre, helps give them a liveliness that is more even and sustained. The wonderfoods in this chapter are, indeed, packed with energy and such nutrients. But they alone will not provide a balanced release. For example, honey is a powerful vitality booster, but it gives a quick energy hit and should be tempered by adding it to protein-, fat-, or fibre-rich foods such as the rye bread and nut butter of the Nutty 'nana' toast (page 36).

The spinach landed in this chapter because of its renowned iron content. Iron is needed for healthy red blood cells to deliver oxygen to each cell in order for it to make energy. So, it's not just a case of fuelling up on quick-release, high energy foods – even the wonderfood ones – but eating them amidst a wide range of foods.

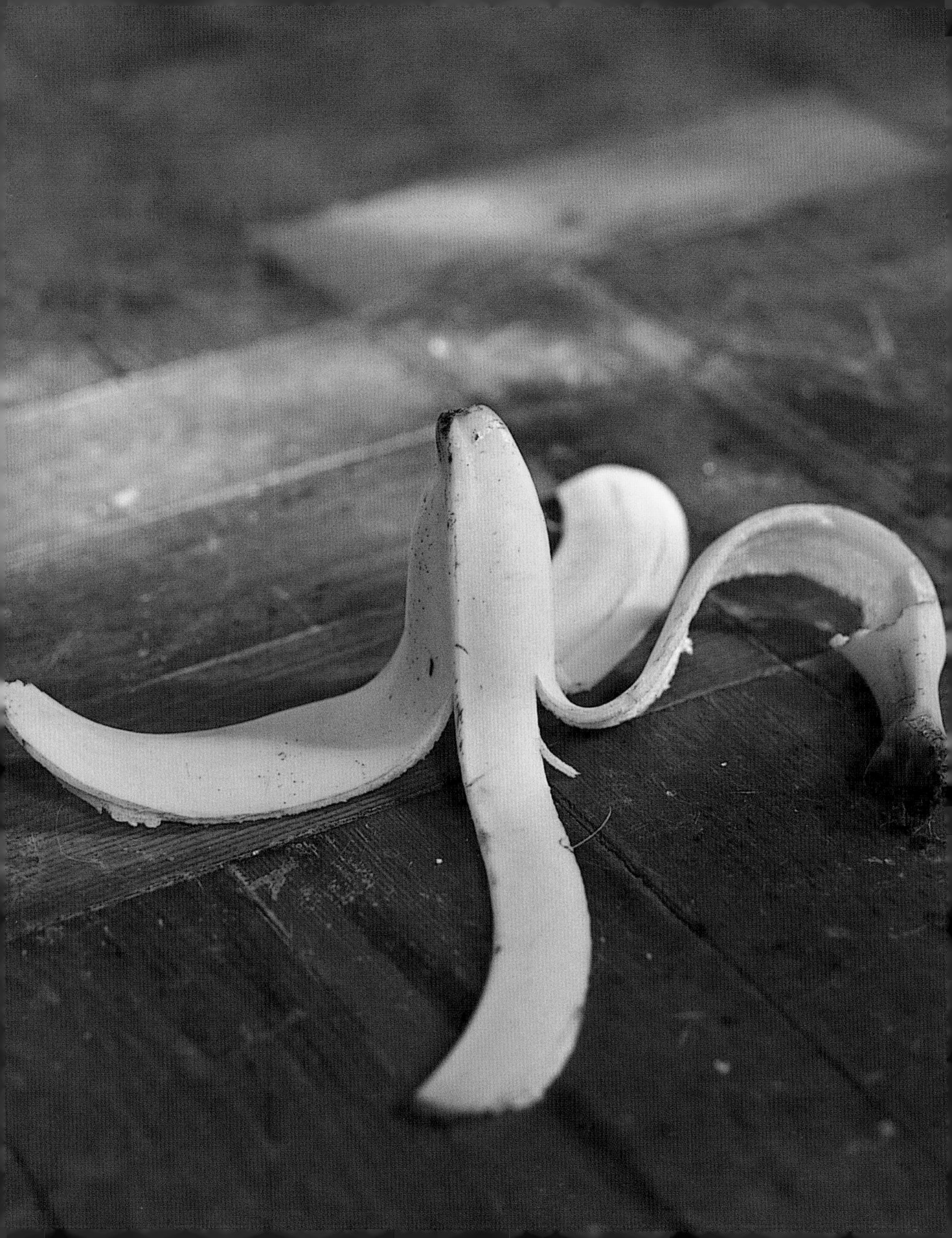

banana

It's a rare child (or adult) who doesn't enjoy a ripe banana that's soft, sweet, portable and energising. It's not just their taste that makes bananas an excellent snack or addition to breakfast – when ripe, the starches they contain will have largely been converted to sugars. This makes them easily digestible, which means the body can readily use the fuel they provide. Eating a banana with some oats, yoghurt or nuts gently slows down the rate at which you actually get the energy from a banana. The easy digestibility of bananas when they are ripe (but not when green) makes them helpful for children with sensitive digestive systems – those who are prone to wind and tummy aches. The soluble fibre, pectin, in bananas also helps soothe the gut. This together with another type of fibre – fructo-oligo-saccharides (FOS) – acts as fuel for the beneficial bacteria in the intestines. Bananas are also a good source of the amino acid, tryptophan, which the body can convert to the calming, good mood hormone, serotonin.

banana passion pots

BANANA AND PASSION FRUIT IS ONE OF MY FAVOURITE FRUIT COMBINATIONS. THESE CREAMY YOGHURT POTS MAKE A GREAT DESSERT FOR CHILDREN. YOU CAN LEAVE OUT THE BLENDING IF YOU PREFER – JUST CHOP THE BANANAS AND TOP THEM WITH THE YOGHURT AND PASSION FRUIT, OMITTING THE VANILLA.

4 small ***bananas****, peeled*
6 tbsp natural ***yoghurt***
1 tsp vanilla extract
2 passion fruit, halved

Cut the bananas into chunks. Whiz them together with the yoghurt and vanilla in a blender, or using a hand-held stick blender. (Older children could do this all themselves and little ones can help plop the banana pieces into a free-standing blender).

Spoon the mixture into four small glasses or pots. Just before eating, scoop the flesh from a passion fruit half on top of each portion.

magic bananas

THIS ISN'T A RECIPE AS SUCH, JUST A MAGICAL WAY OF CUTTING UP BANANAS THAT YOU CAN DO AS A TRICK TO IMPRESS THE CHILDREN – AND ONE THAT THEY CAN LEARN TO DO ON THEIR FRIENDS.

1 ***banana*** *per child*

All of this should be done out of sight of the child(ren): Hold the banana upright and carefully pierce the skin about 2cm from one end with a pin or fine, short skewer, inserting it horizontally as far as the inside of the skin on the other side. Gently swivel the pin horizontally, pivoting from the point at which it went into the skin. What you are, in effect, doing, is cutting across the banana inside its skin, using the pin. Do this again 2cm further down the banana, and continue until you have 'sliced' the whole thing.

Then the moment of magic arrives. With some fanfare in front of the child(ren): with the banana still upright, carefully peel it, strip by strip to reveal a banana that is already sliced even though it's just been peeled before their eyes!

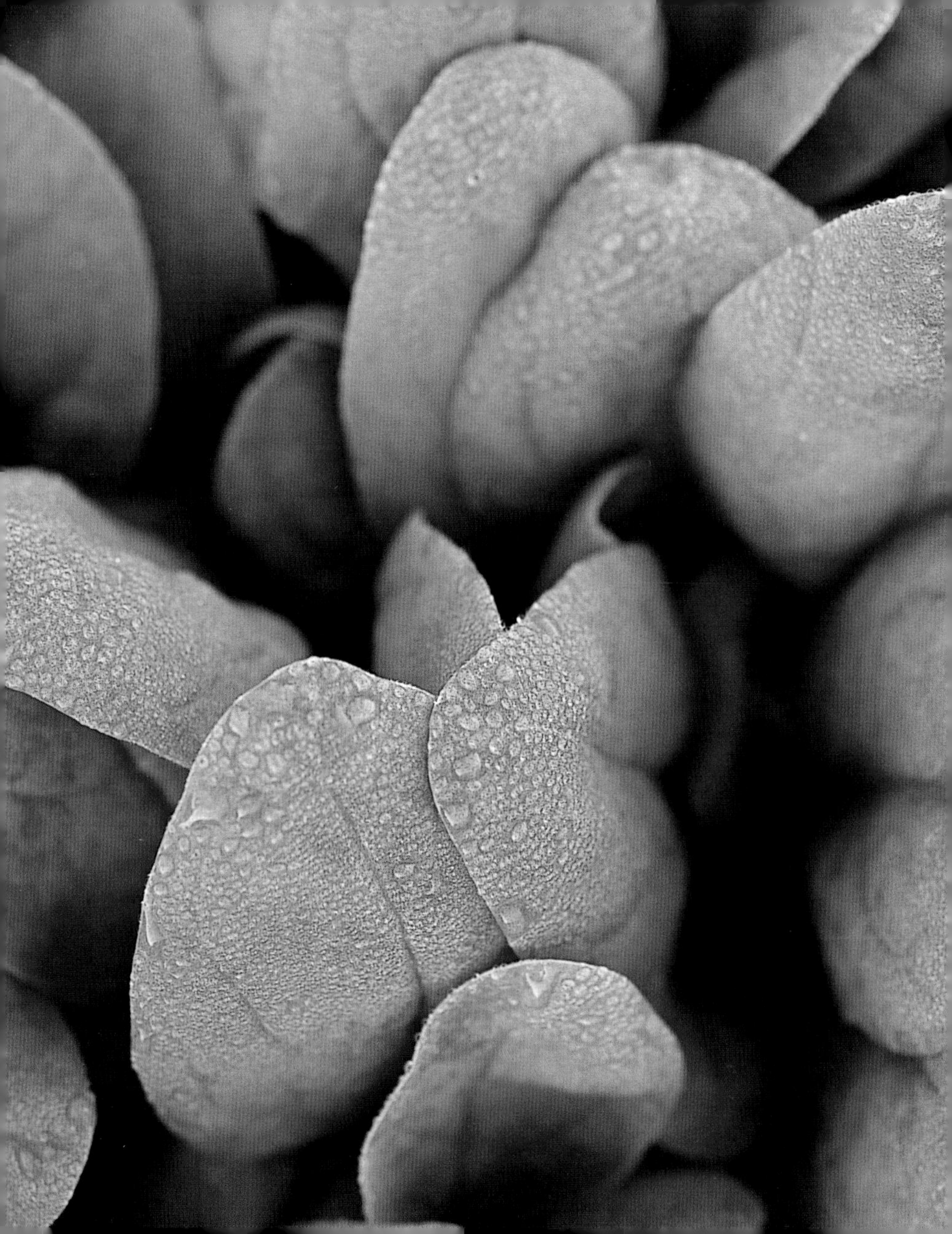

spinach

Let's not kid ourselves, spinach is hardly a big favourite with children and Popeye isn't really around any more to promote its virtues. But this leafy green is such a good, versatile food that it can sell itself. Spinach is best known for its high levels of that vital mineral, iron, which is needed in children particularly for growth, muscle development and by girls as they start menstruating. Iron forms part of the molecule in red blood cells called haemoglobin, which is responsible for carrying oxygen from the lungs to the cells. It is therefore essential for each cell in the body to make energy and this explains why one of the first signs of being low in iron is tiredness. That said, the iron in spinach is not the most absorbable form for humans (compared with the iron in eggs, fish or meat), but eating it with vitamin C rich foods (such as a squeeze of lemon juice) helps increase absorption, which is especially important if your child is vegetarian. Spinach is a good source of folic acid, also needed for proper growth, and vitamin K, which helps with blood clotting and healthy bones.

pond soup

YOU MAY OR MAY NOT PREFER TO INTRODUCE THIS SOUP BY A DIFFERENT NAME, DEPENDING ON YOUR CHILDREN'S FEELINGS ABOUT TADPOLES AND NEWTS. IT FREEZES WELL, SO CONSIDER MAKING DOUBLE AND FREEZING HALF.

1 tbsp olive oil
1 medium ***onion****, peeled and thinly sliced*
1 medium potato, peeled and roughly chopped
2 ***thyme*** *sprigs (or 1 heaped tsp dried thyme)*
1 litre water
500g baby leaf ***spinach***
4 heaped tsp natural ***yoghurt****, to serve*

Heat the olive oil in a large saucepan over a medium heat. Add the onion, potato and thyme, and soften for about 5 minutes.

Pour in the water, stir and bring to the boil, then turn down the heat and simmer gently for 20 minutes.

Add the spinach and stir until the leaves are limp. Turn off the heat and leave the soup to stand for about 10 minutes. Discard the thyme sprigs.

Whiz the soup, using a free-standing or hand-held stick blender, until smooth, then pour into warm bowls. Add a blob of yoghurt to each bowl.

popeye puffs

FOR THESE YOU COULD, OF COURSE, GO TO THE EFFORT OF MAKING PUFF PASTRY, BUT YOU'D HAVE TO LOOK THAT UP IN ANOTHER, MORE SERIOUS, COOKERY BOOK! MAKE THE PUFFS ANY SHAPE YOU LIKE, OR EVEN LEAVE THEM OPEN.

1 tbsp olive oil
2 medium ***onions****, peeled and finely chopped*
2 ***garlic*** *cloves, peeled and crushed*
250g leaf ***spinach****, washed and chopped*
1 ***egg***
200g feta cheese, finely crumbled
1 tbsp ***sunflower seeds***
2 tsp ***lemon*** *juice*
1 tbsp ***mint*** *leaves, finely chopped*
1 tbsp ***parsley*** *leaves, finely chopped*
200g ready-made puff pastry

Preheat the oven to 180°C/Gas 4. Heat the olive oil in a frying pan and soften the onions and garlic over a low heat for about 10 minutes. Add the spinach and stir for about a minute until just wilted. Take off the heat.

Beat the egg lightly in a large bowl. Pour about 1 tbsp into a cup and reserve. Tip the spinach mix into the bowl and toss with the egg. Add the feta, sunflower seeds, lemon juice and herbs; mix well.

Now shape the puffs (small children can help here). Roll out the pastry and cut four squares. Brush the edges with some of the beaten egg.

To make triangular puffs, divide the spinach mix amongst the squares, piling it on to a quarter of each square. Then fold the opposite corner over the filling and press the edges together firmly, pinching to seal them well.

Brush with beaten egg and poke a couple of small holes in the top to allow the steam to escape. Bake for 15–20 minutes until the filling is set and the pastry is golden brown.

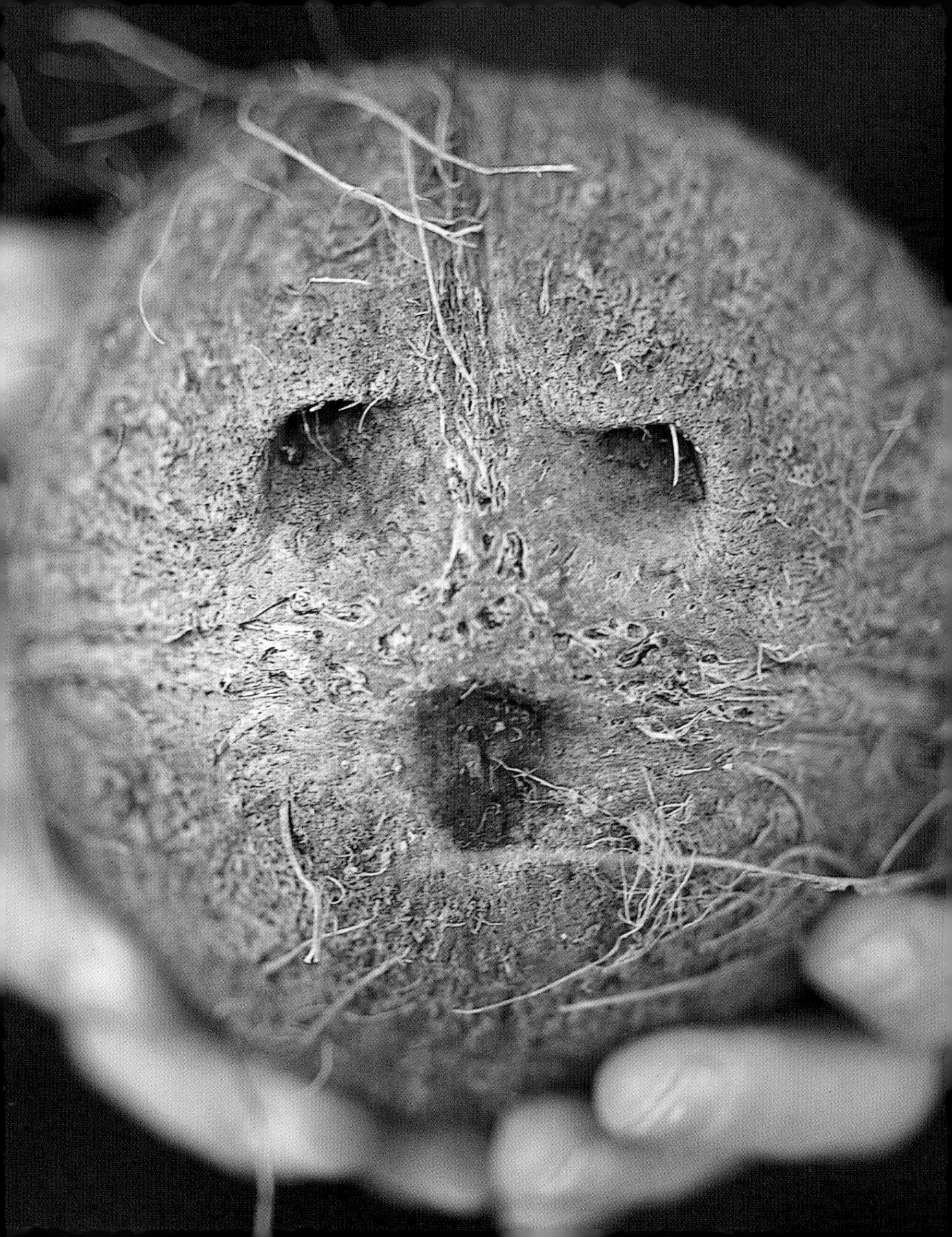

coconut

Long gone are the days when our only exposure to coconuts was at a funfair. The symbol of tropical beaches is increasingly used in our own kitchens in both sweet and savoury dishes. The name comes from the word '*coco*' meaning grinning or monkey face in southern Europe, apparently because the three marks on the shell resemble a face. Coconuts are one of the rare plant foods that contain saturated fats (SF). Although SFs are normally considered undesirable, coconut contains a type called medium chain triglycerides (MCTs), which are easily digested and can help the body make energy. Coconuts also contain other natural substances that the body can use to fight off fungal, viral and bacterial infections. If you're lucky enough to live in a city where Asian grocers sell fresh, green shelled coconuts, do buy them. Your children (and you) can enjoy the cooling, nutritious water inside as a drink – alone or blended with fruits. Then you can scoop the fresh, soft flesh straight from the shell into waiting mouths, or use it as a topping for fruit salad or grilled chicken.

tropical smoothie

THIS MAKES A GREAT BREAKFAST DRINK OR A WONDERFULLY REFRESHING SNACK FOR MID-MORNING OR MID-AFTERNOON. IF YOU CAN'T GET FRESH MANGO OR PINEAPPLE, YOU CAN USE FRUIT CANNED IN NATURAL JUICE.

1 ***mango****, peeled, halved and stoned*
1/2 ***banana****, peeled*
1/4 ***pineapple****, peeled and cored*
2 tbsp ***coconut*** *milk*
4 tbsp natural ***yoghurt***
200ml ***pineapple*** *juice*

Cut the fruit into chunks. Whiz all the ingredients together in a blender, or in a jug using a hand-held stick blender, until smooth. (Small children can help by plopping the ingredients into a free-standing blender.)

Pour into tumblers and serve immediately.

NOTE For a super-enhanced breakfast smoothie, add a splash of hemp or flax (linseed) oil.

coconut veggie stir-fry

AS A CHILD, ANYTHING 'CHINESE' WAS ALWAYS A FAVOURITE IN OUR HOUSE – PERHAPS MADE MORE FUN BY TRYING TO EAT WITH CHOPSTICKS.

2 spring ***onions****, trimmed*
1 ***carrot****, peeled*
4 baby corn
1/2 ***red pepper****, deseeded*
handful of sugarsnap peas or mangetout
large handful of baby ***spinach*** *leaves or kale*
1 tbsp olive oil
1cm piece fresh root ***ginger****, peeled and finely grated*
1 ***garlic*** *clove, peeled and crushed*
3 tbsp cashew ***nuts***
1 tsp Chinese five spice powder (optional)
1 tbsp tamari (or soy sauce), or to taste
100ml ***coconut*** *milk*

Prepare all the vegetables for cooking, aiming to make the pieces all more or less the same size: slice the spring onions; cut the carrot into thin strips; slice the baby corn; cut the red pepper into squares; halve the sugarsnaps; roughly tear the spinach (small children can help here).

Heat a wok or large frying pan and add the olive oil. Add the ginger, garlic and cashew nuts, together with the five spice powder if using, and toss continuously over a medium high heat for about 1 minute.

Add the spring onions, carrot and corn to the wok and toss quickly over the heat for a minute or two, then add all the other vegetables, the tamari and coconut milk. Stir and toss to 'steam-fry' for about 4 minutes.

Serve straight away on a pile of brown rice or rice noodles.

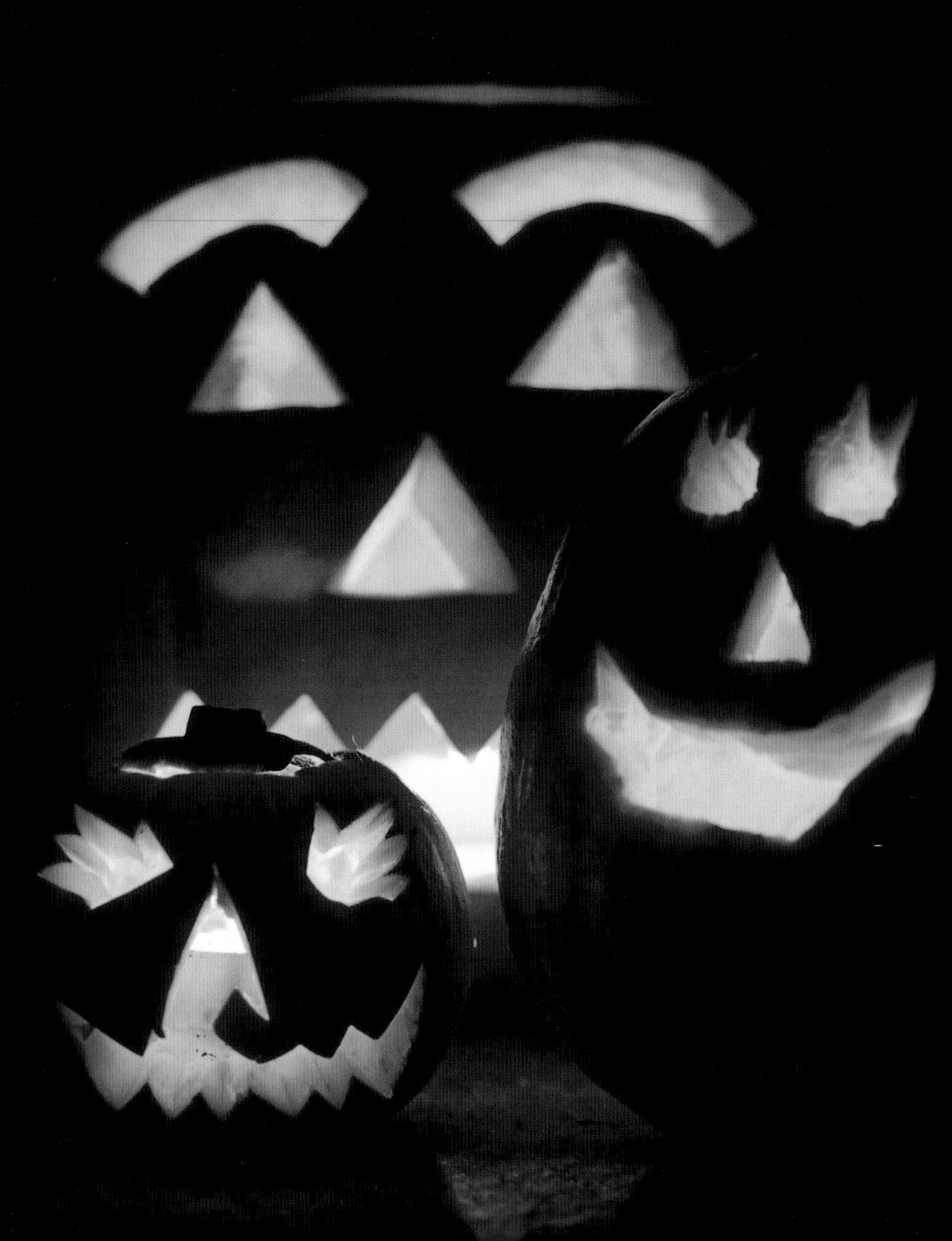

pumpkin & squash

If your children are more accustomed to seeing pumpkins as Hallowe'en lanterns than on their plates, now is a good time to change that. Pumpkins – and other members of the squash family – have a starchy sweetness that appeals to children. This starch makes them a good, high fibre source of slow-releasing energy. Although they do contain a lot of fibre, pumpkins are relatively easy on the digestion and can help relieve constipation. Squash varieties differ in shape, size and colour, although the more orange they are, the higher in beta carotene, the plant form of vitamin A. This is important not only for good skin health but also for our inside skin, such as that lining the intestines and lungs. This makes it a useful food for children with eczema or asthma, or a tendency to frequent coughs. The tough skin gives these vegetables a long shelf-life, so you can always have a butternut (perhaps the most tasty) or other variety sitting on standby in the kitchen. They're remarkably versatile – good slow roasted (even in the skin), mashed, in soup, pies or stews, or as a vessel for other foods.

butternut soup

FOR A VEGETARIAN SOUP – THAT'S ALSO CHEAPER – LEAVE OUT THE PRAWNS AND USE TAMARI INSTEAD OF FISH SAUCE. TEST THE THAI CURRY PASTE OUT YOURSELF FIRST, AS SOME BRANDS ARE WAY TOO HOT FOR CHILDREN... AND SOME ADULTS! THOSE PRODUCED IN THIS COUNTRY (RATHER THAN THAILAND) ARE USUALLY LESS AUTHENTIC AND LESS HOT.

1 large butternut ***squash***
1 tsp olive oil
1 tbsp red Thai curry paste, or to taste
1 medium ***onion****, peeled and finely chopped*
2 ***garlic*** *cloves, peeled and crushed*
800ml vegetable stock
400ml ***coconut*** *milk*
2 tbsp Thai fish sauce
2–3 medium large raw prawns per person, shelled and deveined (optional)
torn ***mint*** *and* ***coriander*** *leaves, to serve*

Halve the squash, scoop out the seeds and peel away the skin, then cut the flesh into cubes.

Heat the olive oil in a large saucepan, add the curry paste and fry, stirring, over a medium heat for a minute. Toss in the onion and garlic and cook for another minute or so, stirring frequently.

Then add the squash, stock, coconut milk and fish sauce, stirring well. Bring to the boil, lower the heat and leave to simmer for about 10 minutes or until the pumpkin is just tender.

About 3 minutes before serving, throw in the prawns and continue to simmer the soup until they turn pink, indicating that they are cooked.

Ladle the soup into warm bowls and add a sprinkling of torn mint and coriander to serve.

butternut boats

THE TOMATO SAUCE HERE HAS LOTS OF USES SO YOU MIGHT LIKE TO MAKE A TRIPLE BATCH AND FREEZE TWO-THIRDS, OR KEEP IN THE FRIDGE AND USE AS THE BASE FOR A PASTA SAUCE OR SOUP THE FOLLOWING DAY.

2 small-medium butternut ***squashes***
olive oil, for rubbing
freshly ground black pepper
FOR THE TOMATO SAUCE
small handful of dried ***shiitake mushrooms***
5 ***tomatoes*** *(or a small 230g can)*
1 tbsp olive oil
1 medium ***onion****, peeled and roughly diced*
2 ***garlic*** *cloves, peeled and crushed*
½ tsp ***thyme*** *leaves*
100g feta cheese, roughly crumbled

Preheat the oven to 190°C/Gas 5. Halve the squashes lengthways and scoop out the seeds. Place skin side down on a baking tray, rub with olive oil, grind pepper over them and put into the oven to bake for about 40 minutes until tender. Meanwhile, make the tomato sauce. Put the mushrooms into a small bowl, pour a little boiling water over to rehydrate them and set aside. If using fresh tomatoes and (like me) you can't bear the skins, drop them into a pan of boiling water for a minute, take out, peel and chop roughly.

Heat the olive oil in a saucepan and soften the onion and garlic with the thyme for 4–5 minutes. Add the tomatoes and the mushrooms with their soaking water. Leave this to simmer very gently until the squash is cooked.

When the squash is ready, spoon some of the tomato sauce into the hollows, top with the feta cheese and return to the oven for 5 minutes. Serve topped with more sauce if you like, alongside a green salad or steamed broccoli.

squish squash

THIS TASTY MASH IS BEST EATEN AS A SIDE DISH TO STICKY CHICKEN (PAGE 153), GRILLED CHICKEN OR A CHICKPEA STEW.

1 large butternut ***squash***
1 medium ***onion****, peeled and diced*
1 tbsp butter
½ tsp ground ***ginger***

Halve the squash lengthways and scoop out the seeds, then peel and roughly dice the flesh. Put into a saucepan with the onion, add water to cover and boil until the squash is soft, about 20 minutes depending on the size of the pieces.

Drain well and return the squash and onion to the pan. Add the butter and ginger and squish it all together with a masher. (Young children can help with the 'squishing'.) Serve hot.

sweet squash with apple stuffing

YOU'RE BEST OFF USING A SMALL, ROUNDISH TYPE OF SQUASH FOR THIS RECIPE. IT MAKES A PRETTY HEFTY DESSERT OR A SUBSTANTIAL TEATIME TREAT, ESPECIALLY IF YOU ADD A LITTLE YOGHURT OR AN INDULGENT SCOOP OF VANILLA ICE CREAM.

2 small-medium ***squashes****, such as acorn squash*
1 tbsp runny ***honey****, plus extra for rubbing*
2 small-medium ***apples***
100ml ***apple*** *juice*
6 ***cardamom*** *pods*
1 ***cinnamon*** *stick*
50g ***raisins***
50g dried ***apricots****, roughly chopped*
12–15 pecan ***nuts****, roughly broken*

Preheat the oven to 190°C/Gas 5. Halve the squashes and remove the seeds, then scoop out some of the flesh, leaving a layer about 1cm thick inside the skin.

Put the squash halves, hollow side up, on a baking tray and rub the flesh with a little honey. Bake in the oven for about 30 minutes depending on size.

Meanwhile, core and roughly chop the apples. Put them into a saucepan with the scooped-out squash, honey, apple juice, spices and dried fruit. (Young children can help simply by putting these ingredients into the pan.) Cover and simmer very gently over a low heat for about 15 minutes. Turn off the heat, leaving the pan covered.

To test whether the squashes are ready, pierce with a fine skewer; they should feel soft. Put a squash half on each plate and spoon the apple mix into the middle. Top with the pecan nuts and serve warm.

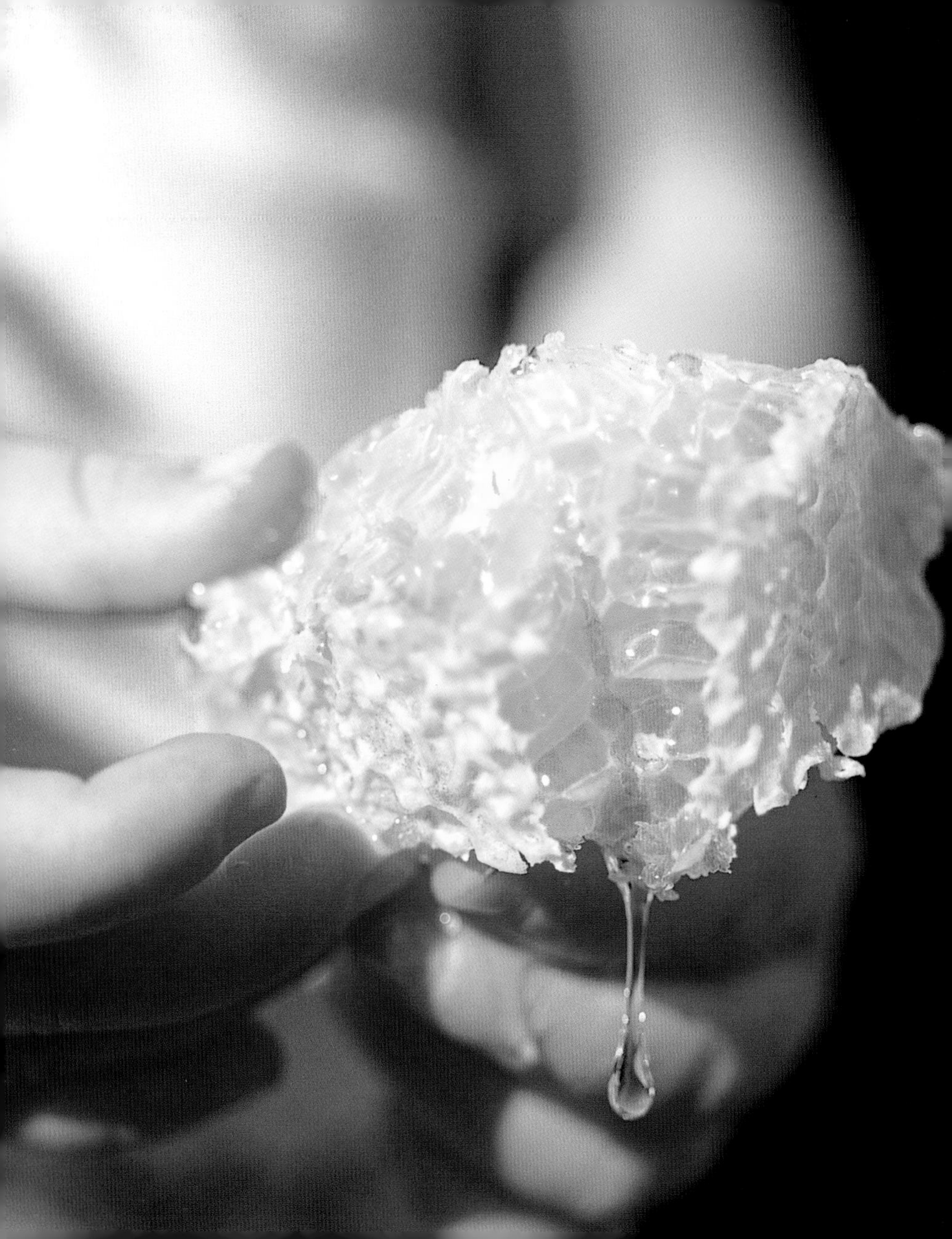

honey

Honey has a wonderful flavour and because it is a relatively nutritious sweetener it's a great way of adding sweetness to children's foods – from wholegrain breakfast cereals to tart fruits and cakes. Bees make honey from nectar for energy food, and for children too, this wonderfood is a rapidly absorbed source of fuel. As such, it is best used in moderation – to avoid the highs and subsequent lows in energy and concentration, the tooth decay and weight gain linked to frequent sugar hits. Not all honeys are equal – many of the blended, cheaper versions sold in supermarkets lack the 'magical' properties that make up about 3% of the pure, raw honeys produced by conscientious beekeepers (the other 97% is sugar). Some of those qualities depend on the flowers from which the bees gathered their nectar; thyme honey, for example, takes on some of the antiseptic characteristics of the plant. Traces of the powerful antiseptic, propolis, which bees make are also found in honey – making it a good addition to a hot drink for a child with a sore throat.

nutty 'nana' toast

THIS IS A DELICIOUS, SATISFYING BREAKFAST OR AFTERNOON TEA.

4 slices of ***rye*** *bread*
4 tsp ***hazelnut*** *or* ***almond*** *butter*
1 ripe ***banana****, thinly sliced*
4 tsp runny ***honey***

Put the grill on to heat. Toast the bread on both sides, then spread it with the nut butter. Arrange the banana slices on the pieces of toast and drizzle honey over the top (children can do this). Put the slices under the grill for 3–4 minutes. Then serve immediately, cut into slices.

sweet & sour chicken

THIS IS A POPULAR DISH WITH CHILDREN – LITTLE ONES CAN HELP WITH COATING THE CHICKEN PIECES. IT GOES WELL WITH SOME STEAMED OR STIR-FRIED CHINESE CABBAGE OR BROCCOLI AND RICE NOODLES.

500g boneless ***chicken*** *breasts, skinned*
2 tbsp olive oil
1 tsp Chinese five spice powder (optional)
½ cm piece fresh root ***ginger****, peeled and grated*
1 ***garlic*** *clove, peeled and crushed*
2 spring ***onions****, trimmed and finely sliced*
¼ ***pineapple****, peeled and diced*
1 tbsp tamari (or soy sauce)
2 tbsp runny ***honey***
2 tbsp ***lime*** *juice*
1 tbsp ***sesame seeds***
120ml ***apple*** *or* ***pineapple*** *juice*

Slice the chicken breasts into strips (not much larger than your little finger). Heat the olive oil in a frying pan, then add the chicken strips with the five spice powder. Squash them down gently with a fish slice and leave them cooking for a couple of minutes until they're a little crispy on the bottom. Then turn them over to do the same on the other side. When the chicken is cooked (cut a piece open to check), remove from the pan with a slotted spoon and lay on kitchen paper to drain.

Put all the remaining ingredients into the frying pan and stir continuously over the heat for 3 or 4 minutes, as the liquid reduces a little.

Tip the chicken back into the pan and heat through in the sauce for a couple of minutes. Serve in warm bowls or plates.

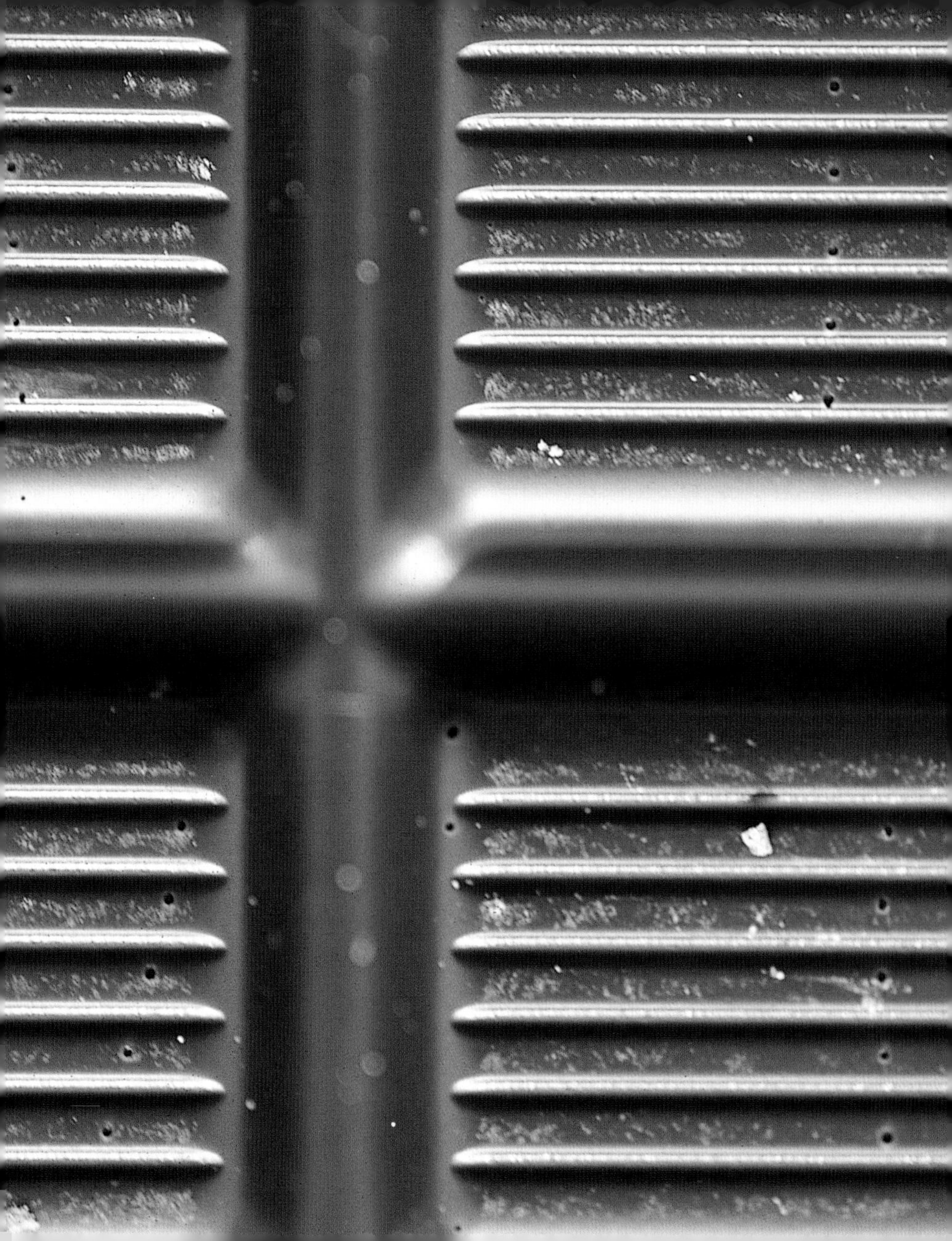

chocolate

The Aztecs in Mexico once used cocoa beans as currency and, to this day, one of their key derivatives – chocolate – is loved by most children. Classifying chocolate as a wonderfood does, as you may suspect, have conditions attached. It is the cocoa itself that has healthy powers. Most chocolate on the market is high in sugar and/or unhealthy, hydrogenated fats but low in cocoa so it doesn't qualify. Be aware, also, that high cocoa chocolate contains stimulants, including caffeine, so should be eaten in small amounts. Even the finest, organic chocolates contain some sugar, which is acceptable once in a while amidst a healthy diet. Apart from its 'soulfood' value, chocolate earns its wonderfood status because scientists have, in the last few years, found powerful antioxidants in cocoa. These are linked to lowering inflammation – useful for keeping blood and blood vessels healthy, and for conditions such as asthma and eczema. Interestingly, two stimulants in cocoa, theobromine and theophylline, are used medically, to relieve lung spasms in asthma and coughs.

fruity chocolate shake

THIS IS SO UNBELIEVABLY DELICIOUS – YOUR CHILDREN MAY EVEN THINK THEY'RE DRINKING A WICKED, RICH, ICE CREAM SHAKE.

2 ripe ***bananas****, peeled*
1 generous tbsp ***cocoa*** *powder*
½ tsp vanilla extract
1 tsp ***honey***
4 heaped tbsp natural ***yoghurt***
150ml ***apple*** *juice*
150ml milk (or ***soya*** *milk or rice milk)*
3–4 ice cubes

Whiz all the ingredients together in a blender and serve immediately.

chocolate apples

THESE ARE IDEAL FOR HALLOWE'EN, BUT YOU DON'T HAVE TO KEEP THEM TO A ONCE-A-YEAR TREAT.

4 medium ***apples***
200g dark ***chocolate****,*
broken into pieces
200g white chocolate,
broken into pieces
TO ASSEMBLE
4 ice lolly sticks

Wash and dry the apples and remove their stalks.

Melt each type of chocolate separately in a heatproof bowl balanced over a saucepan of gently simmering water (do not let the water come into contact with the bowl otherwise the chocolate might seize). When the chocolate has almost all melted, stir until smooth.

Push a lolly stick into the top of each apple, to use as a handle. Take the bowls of melted chocolate off the pans. Now it's time to coat the apples (young children can help here.) Dip the apples into the dark chocolate, using a spoon to dribble chocolate into tricky areas. Then drizzle some white chocolate over the dark layer, using another spoon.

Lay the apples on a tray covered with non-stick parchment and put them into the fridge for about an hour to set.

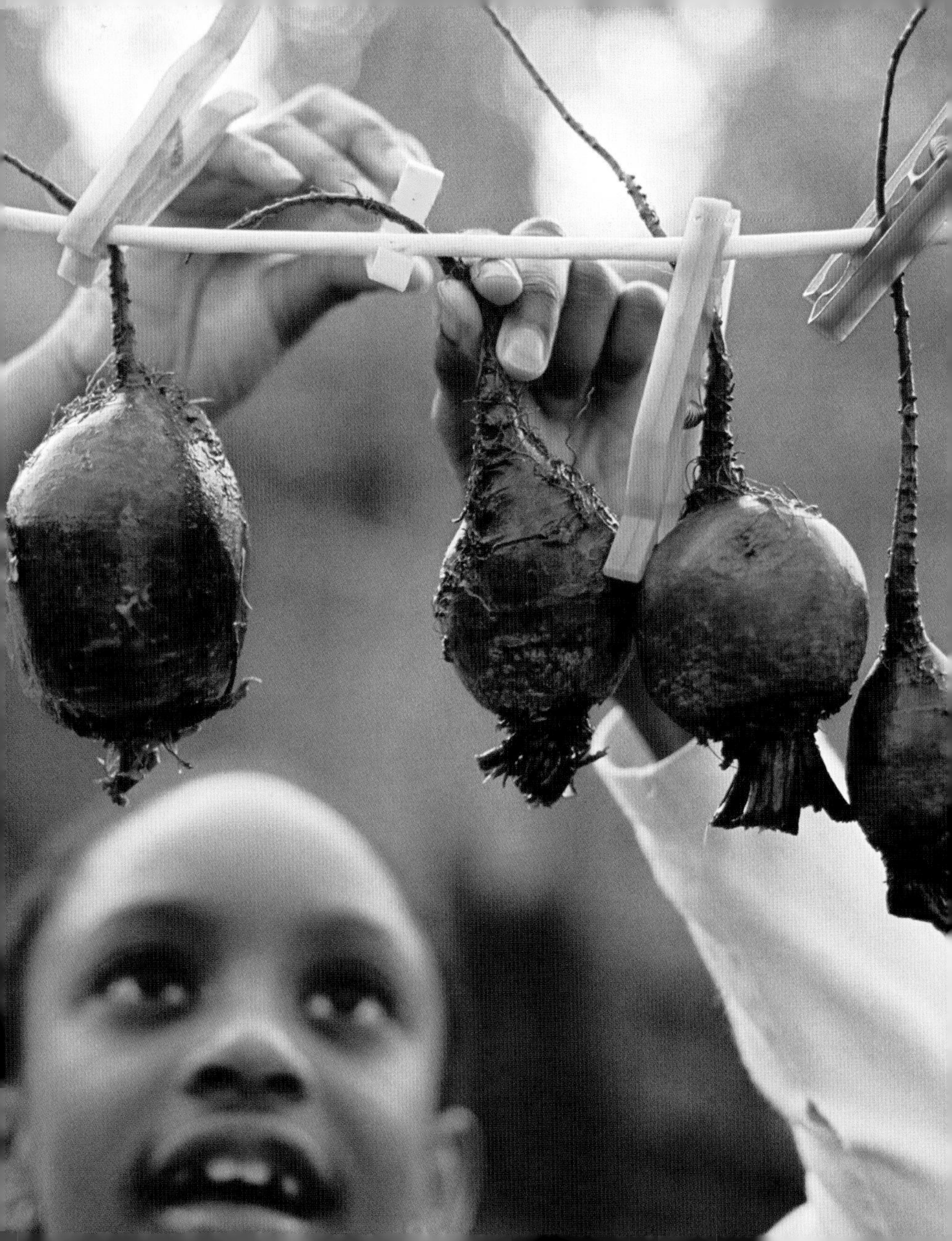

beetroot

The official family name of beetroot is 'goosefoot' – referring to its leaves rather than anything to do with a feathery bird. At one time, only the leaves were eaten as food, the roots saved for their medicinal properties. Not that health value will encourage children to eat anything, so let beetroot sell itself with its buttery sweetness and enticing colour. It's the ghastly acidic pickled ones that put most children off. The sweet taste of fresh beetroot reflects its relatively high sugar content, which is a source of energy, packaged with a good dose of gentle fibre and nutrients. The fibre and generally detoxifying nature makes beetroot a good tonic for the digestive system as well as the liver. It is never too early to consider the role of wonderfoods in protecting against heart disease and cancer, and beetroot contains natural chemicals that help do just that. Their powerful antioxidants work hard behind the scenes in the liver and throughout the body to boost the immune system. Beetroot are particularly high in folic acid, the B vitamin needed for, amongst other things, proper growth and development.

sweet purple filling

ONLY NATURE COULD MAKE SUCH A SPECTACULAR COLOUR. THIS MUSH GOES WONDERFULLY IN A SANDWICH, ON CRACKERS, OR PILED ON TO JACKET POTATOES.

*3 medium **beetroots**, trimmed and scrubbed*
splash of olive oil
freshly ground black pepper
200g cottage cheese with chives
*2 tsp **lemon** juice*
pinch of sea salt
*1 tbsp chopped **parsley***

Preheat the oven to 190°C/Gas 5 and line an ovenproof tray with baking paper. Cut the beetroot into 2–3cm cubes and spread out on the lined tray. Splash with a little olive oil, grind over some pepper and toss to mix. Bake in the oven for about 30–40 minutes until the beetroot is soft (enough to mash with a fork).

Tip into a bowl and leave to cool, then mash with the cottage cheese, lemon juice, salt and parsley. (Children can help with the mashing.)

Use as a sandwich filling or spread, or to top hot jacket potatoes.

sweet roast veg

THESE GO DOWN SO WELL, YOU MAY WANT TO MAKE DOUBLE FOR SECONDS OR TO EAT THE NEXT DAY.

1 medium ***sweet potato****,*
scrubbed
2 medium ***beetroots****,*
trimmed and scrubbed
1 ***red pepper****, halved, cored and deseeded*
splash of olive oil
2–3 ***thyme*** *sprigs, or 1 tsp dried thyme*
freshly ground black pepper

Preheat the oven to 190°C/Gas 5. Slice the sweet potato into 1.5cm thick rounds and the beetroots into slightly thinner 1cm thick rounds. Cut the red pepper into strips.

Place all the veggies on a baking tray – ideally lined with greaseproof paper to prevent them from sticking (and make washing up easier). Drizzle the veggies with olive oil, sprinkle with the thyme and season with pepper. Give them a good shake to coat well (small children can help here).

Bake in the oven for about 30 minutes until the veggies are cooked through – prick with a skewer to check that they feel soft.

Serve with meat, fish or poultry, such as Lemon roast chicken (page 221).

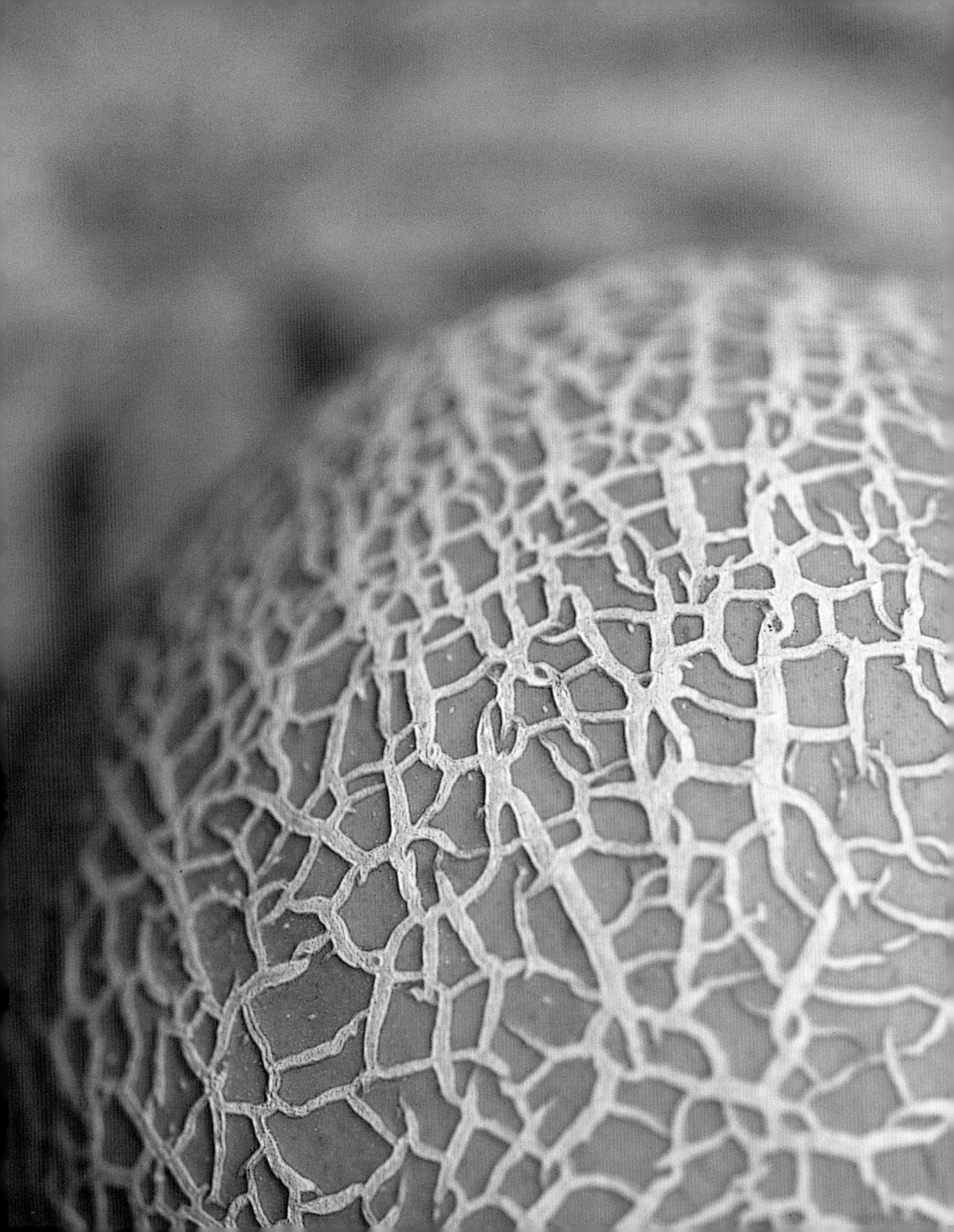

watermelon & melon

Most children like melons, and find the colour, crunch and thirst-quenching nature of watermelons particularly appealing. It so happens that they load children up with important nutrients too. Not least of their benefits is water. In arid areas of the world, watermelons are prized for their high water content, which makes them not only hydrating but also cleansing. Within that water is diluted natural sugar, which can be turned into energy in the body. The red flesh of watermelons and orange melons indicates their rich content of carotenoids, such as beta carotene and lycopene, which are needed for the defence system and healthy skin, eyes and lungs. They both also contain vitamin C, famous for boosting immunity. Their flesh is digested very rapidly but only when they land in an empty stomach, so they're best eaten alone. Blend watermelon flesh, seeds and all, to make a thick, refreshing drink, for your children and they will also get the nutrients that hide inside the seeds such as zinc, which is used for growth and immunity.

chicken salad in a melon

THIS MAKES A LOVELY SUMMER WEEKEND LUNCH FOR EVERYONE. THE POMEGRANATE IS A GORGEOUS EXTRA IF YOU CAN FIND THEM IN THE SHOPS.

2 ***melons****, such as Cantaloupe or Galia*
2 tbsp natural ***yoghurt***
1 tbsp ***lime*** *juice*
1 tbsp tamari (or soy sauce)
1 tbsp runny ***honey***
2 cooked ***chicken*** *breasts, roughly diced*
1 medium ***pomegranate****, seeds only*

Cut the melons in half across the middle – in a zigzag fashion if you like – and scoop out the seeds. Then, using a curved grapefruit knife (if you have one), cut the flesh from the skin. Cut the melon flesh into bite-sized chunks.

Young children can help now. In a large bowl, mix the yoghurt with the lime juice, tamari and honey. Add the melon and chicken and toss it all well together.

Spoon the salad back into the melon skins. Top each portion with some pomegranate seeds just before serving.

watermelon slurpie

THIS IS A GREAT, COOLING 'SLUSH' IN THE SUMMER.

8 big, ripe hunks of ***watermelon***
handful of ice cubes

Remove the skin from the watermelon but don't bother to take out the seeds from the flesh as they are packed with vitamins and minerals. Whiz up the ice and fruit in a blender, pour into tumblers and serve immediately.

spit the pip

OK, SO THIS ISN'T REALLY A RECIPE, BUT IT'S GREAT FUN, ESPECIALLY ON THE BEACH OR ROUND THE PADDLING POOL. SOME MAY SAY 'DISGUSTING' BUT PERHAPS THAT'S THE SORT OF CHILD I WAS!

1 ripe ***watermelon***

Cut the watermelon into 'U' shaped slices and hand one to each child... and playful adults who don't mind getting a bit sticky! (Swimsuits are the best attire.)

Each child eats their watermelon, saving the pips of each mouthful in their cheek to play. Then the real fun starts: see who can spit the pips the furthest or, for extra mess and stickiness, at each other!

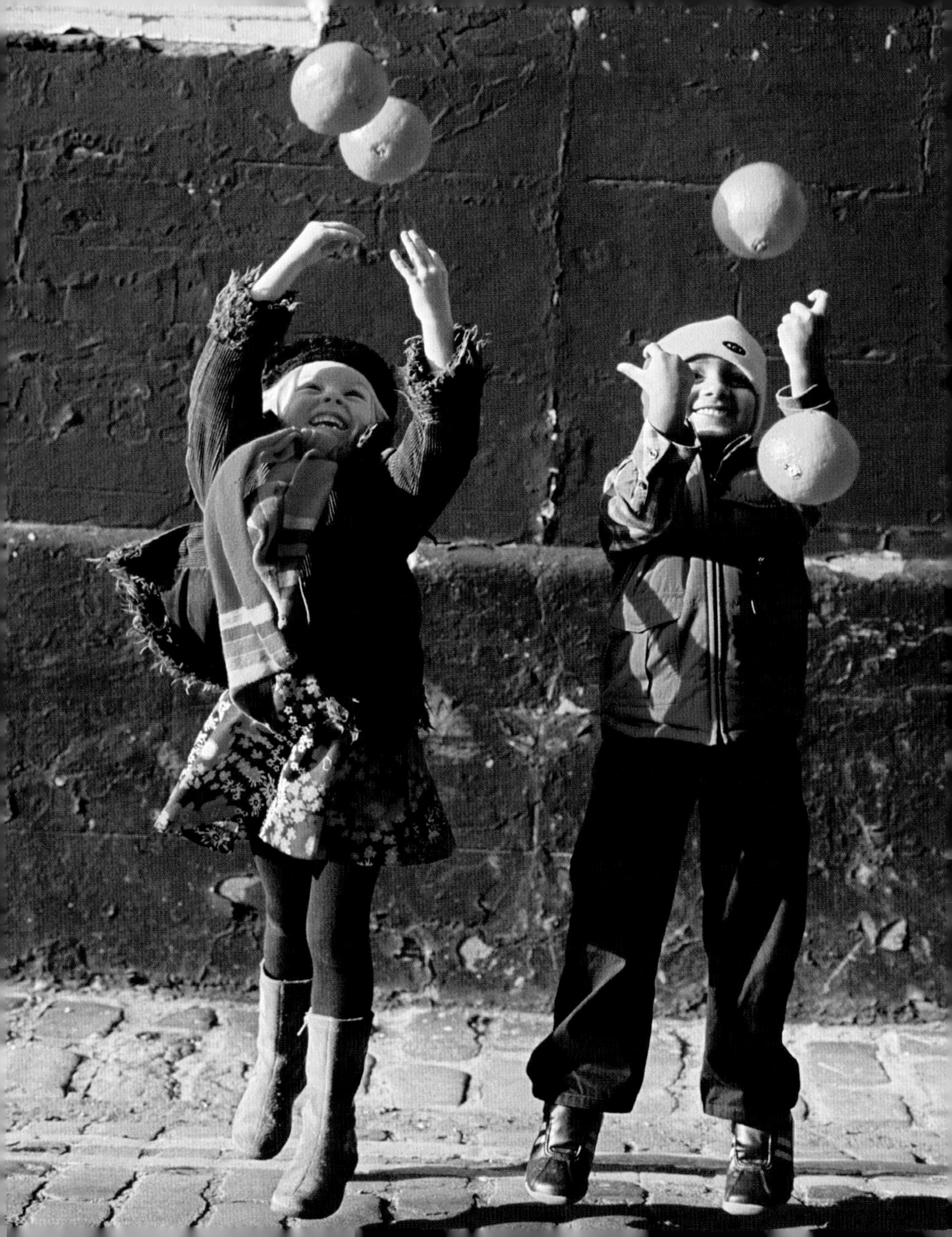

orange

In one form or another – as juicy jaffas, satsumas, tangerines or as juice – oranges are the world's favourite fruit. It is best, of course, to give your children the whole fruit, so they not only get all the vitamins and minerals, but also the fibre. Freshly squeezed juice is good too – in effect, a predigested source of high energy and minerals that encourage movement in the gut, alongside other vital nutrients. Orange's renowned vitamin C content is best derived from eating the fruit or freshly pressed juice, as it is unstable and can be lost during processing and storage. Vitamin C is, though, just one of an orange's powerful defence-boosting antioxidants. Others are citrus flavonoids called hesperetin, naringenin and herperidin. Between them, these antioxidants have been shown to protect against heart disease, cancer and inflammation generally. Some are found mainly in the pith, so when you peel an orange for your child, don't be too particular about taking it all off. Other natural chemicals in oranges, called polyphenols are antiviral and anti-allergenic, while the folic acid is crucial for proper growth.

orangey carrot and lentil soup

ORANGE JUICE LENDS A LOVELY SWEETNESS AND A THIRD ORANGE HUE TO THIS THICK, WARMING SOUP.

*100g **orange** lentils*
1 tbsp olive oil
*1 medium **onion**, peeled and finely diced*
1 level tsp ground cumin
*2 large **carrots**, peeled and chopped*
*230g can chopped **tomatoes**, or 3–4 fresh ones*
*juice of 2 large **oranges***
*1 tsp grated **orange** zest*
pinch of sea salt
700ml vegetable stock

Wash the lentils thoroughly in a sieve, checking for and removing any grit.

Heat the olive oil in a large saucepan and soften the onion with the cumin for about 10 minutes. Add the carrots and lentils, stir for another minute, then put in the rest of the ingredients. Bring to the boil, cover and simmer for about 30 minutes.

Allow the soup to cool a little, then whiz using a hand-held stick blender until quite smooth and thick. Just add a little more boiling water as you blend it if you want the soup to be a bit thinner.

japanese orange dragons

MY FATHER ONCE RETURNED FROM A BUSINESS TRIP TO JAPAN WITH THIS WAY OF CUTTING UP ORANGES, HAVING LEARNED IT FROM THE JAPANESE MAN SITTING NEXT TO HIM ON THE PLANE. IT MAKES EATING AN ORANGE SO MUCH MORE FUN.

4 small, juicy ***oranges***

Lay the orange on a board with the stalk and base facing to the sides. Using a sharp knife, cut the orange across the segments into generous rounds.

Then, take a slice and at a point between two segments, carefully cut through the skin and as far as the centre of the slice. Carefully prise open the slice, separating the little triangular segments: you end up with a flat line of orange skin with a series of little triangles poking out from it – the dragon fins. Repeat with the other slices.

This is much easier to do than to describe in words – so give it a go and you'll find your children will be keener to eat the oranges than if they'd had to peel them in the usual way.

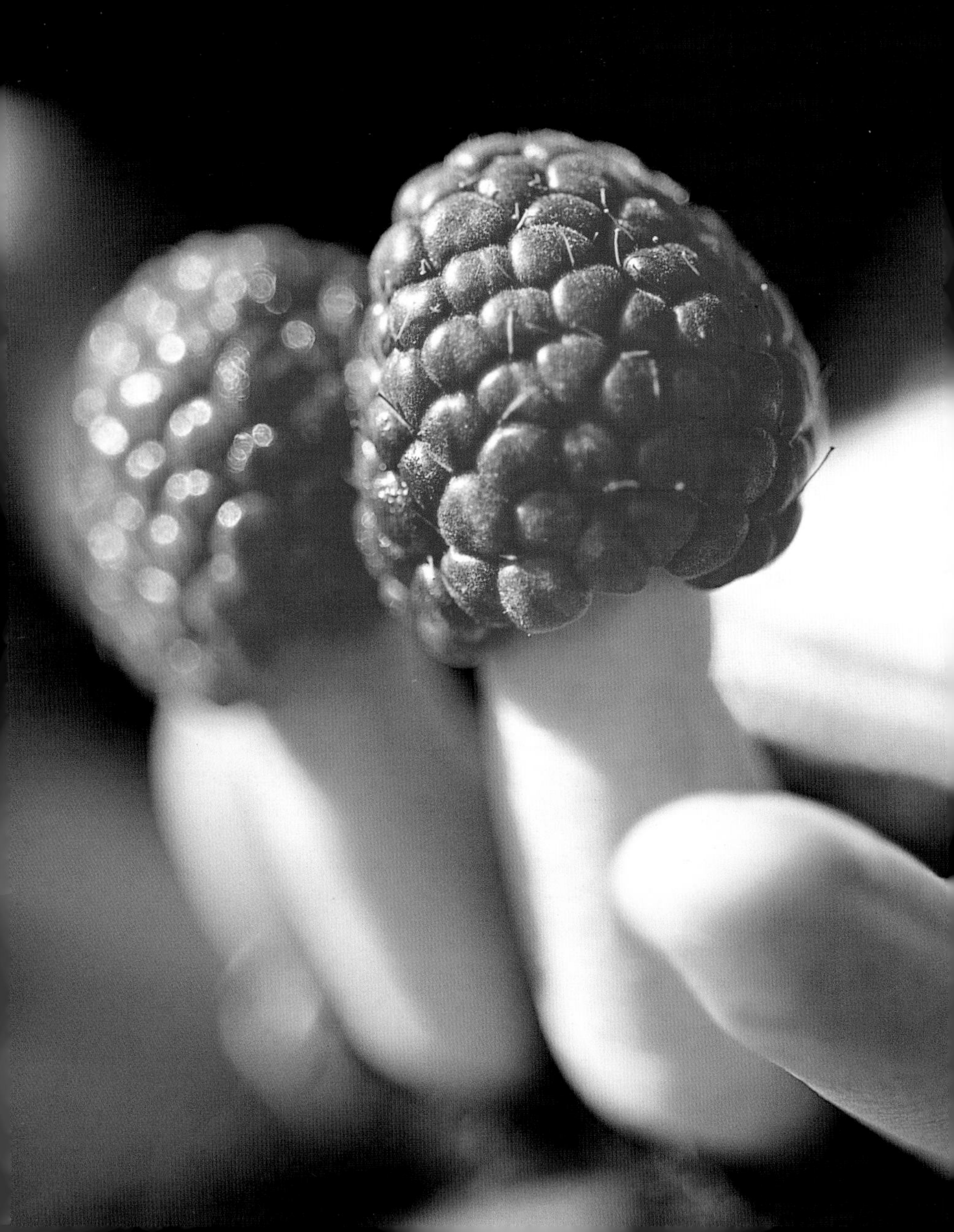

raspberries

Raspberries are related to roses, as their thorns suggest, but they are even closer cousins to blackberries, and their hybrids, loganberries and boysenberries. They are one of the most nutritious berries, so it's worth indulging in their preciously short season. Raspberries are one of the richest sources of a tannin called ellagic acid. This substance is fast gaining a reputation as a powerful antioxidant that not only helps protect against the development of cancerous cells, but generally supports the immune system. Other phytonutrients, quercetin and several anthocyanins that give raspberries their glorious red colour, have similarly protective qualities. Although not usually the sweetest of berries, they are an easily digestible source of energy that most children love. Little will they know that they are consuming wonderful doses of such important nutrients, plus manganese, vitamin C and others. Manganese works to fire one of the body's own antioxidant enzymes, but it is also essential for healthy skin, bone and cartilage, as well as processing glucose to make energy.

salad of baby greens with raspberries

YOU MIGHT THINK THIS IS QUITE A SOPHISTICATED SALAD FOR CHILDREN BUT THE RASPBERRIES AND SWEET DRESSING USUALLY MAKE IT POPULAR. IT CAN BE EATEN WITH ANY FISH, MEAT OR POULTRY SUCH AS THE LAMB BURGERS (PAGE 126) OR BAKED TURKEY ROLLS (PAGE 152).

250g mixed baby ***spinach*** *and lettuce leaves, washed*
1 ***avocado***
200g ***raspberries***
16 ***almonds****, roughly chopped*

FOR THE DRESSING
50g ***raspberries***
2 tbsp ***walnut*** *oil (or* ***sesame*** *oil)*
1 tbsp cider vinegar
1 tbsp ***apple*** *juice*
1 tsp runny ***honey***

First, make the dressing. Whiz the ingredients together in a small bowl, using a hand-held stick blender, until smooth.

Put the spinach and lettuce leaves into a large bowl. Halve, peel and dice the avocado and add to the salad leaves with the raspberries. Drizzle the dressing over and toss gently to mix.

Divide the salad among four plates and scatter the chopped almonds on top.

raspberry brûlée

THIS IS A HEALTHY, YET STILL SCRUMPTIOUS VERSION OF THE TRULY RICH CRÈME BRÛLÉE. YOU CAN USE FROZEN RASPBERRIES INSTEAD OF FRESH ONES IF YOU LIKE.

250g ***raspberries***
300ml Greek-style natural ***yoghurt***
1 ripe ***banana***
1 tsp vanilla extract
1 tbsp runny ***honey***
2 tsp brown or caster sugar

Put three or four raspberries in the bottom of each of four small ramekins or heatproof glass dishes.

Put the rest of the raspberries into a bowl and add the yoghurt, banana, vanilla and honey. Whiz to combine, using a hand-held stick blender.

Pour the yoghurt mix over the raspberries in the ramekins and put them in the fridge to chill.

Just before serving, sprinkle a layer of sugar over the top and glaze with a cook's blow-torch or under a hot grill until the sugar has caramelised. Leave to cool and set before eating.

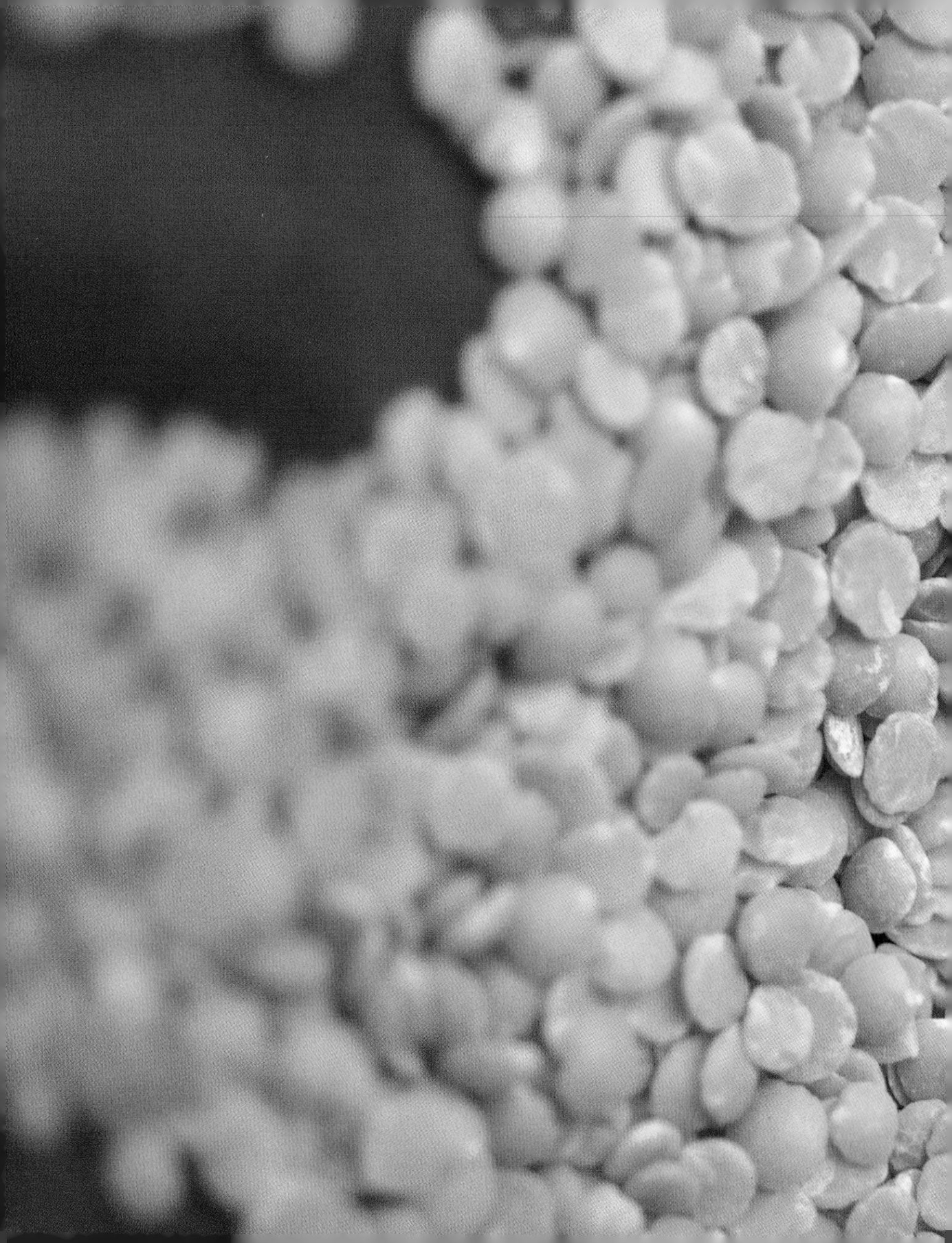

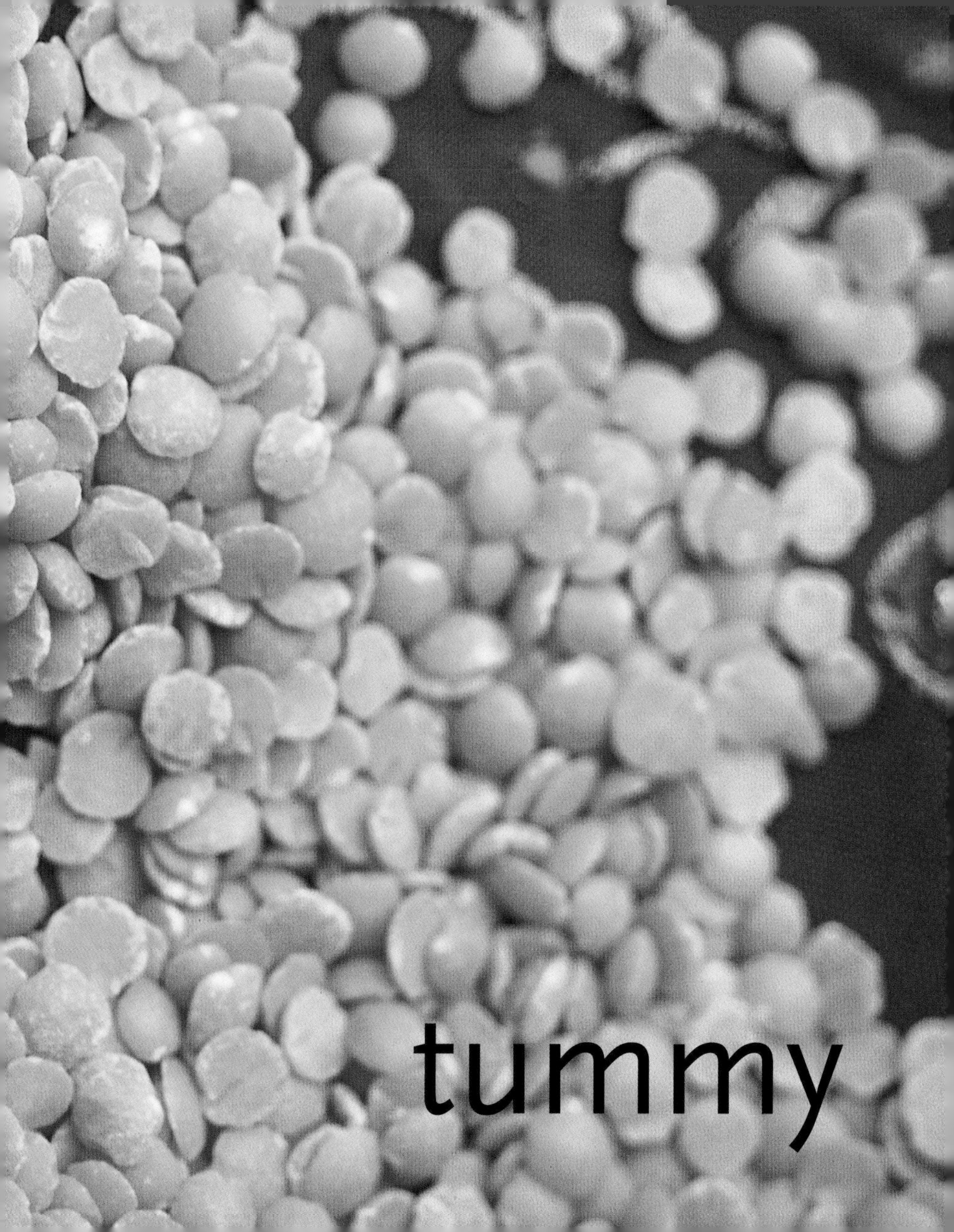

tummy

"I've got tummy ache" is one excuse for getting off school that nobody can really question. Tummy aches are invisible and have a myriad of possible causes. Tummies – in fact the entire length of the gastrointestinal tract – are not only complex tubes with many different roles along the way, but they also have to deal with 'foreign' substances in the form of food several times a day. It's par for the course for babies to be sick from time to time as they get used to different foods, but even older children are susceptible to all sorts of digestive troubles.

Good digestion begins even before food enters the mouth – with the foods you choose to eat. Opting to feed your children the wonderfoods in this book is a great place to start. Quirks, allergies and genetics aside, our guts benefit if we eat mainly these foods and keep sweet, stodgy, fatty, highly processed, additive-laden foods to a minimum. That said, it is important to encourage children to take time over food, to pause between mouthfuls and not to race through meals. This way they are more likely to chew properly, breaking up the food and mixing it well with saliva... and so begins good digestion.

Tummy usually refers to any area below the chest, but strictly speaking, the stomach is the organ into which food goes once it's just been swallowed. If food arrives there poorly chewed, the stomach – and later the intestines – have a much harder job of breaking it down. Anxiety also interferes with digestion. When we are stressed, and it's easy to forget that children can be, our guts are inefficient. Of course, we need to carry on eating when we are anxious, but it's worth bearing in mind that simpler meals and healthy ingredients are easier on the gut, and good for helping the body cope at hard times. Apples, especially cooked, are light on digestion, and pineapple contains enzymes that help break down food.

A common digestive disorder in children is constipation. Many of the foods in this section, as throughout the book, are naturally high in fibre, which helps bulk out the stool, making its movement along the intestines and ultimately out of the body much easier. For fibre to be of much use, it's essential that children have enough fluids, particularly water or watered down fruit juices. Without sufficient water, the body draws more liquid out of the stool, making it hard, compacted and difficult to pass.

Even if a child is not constipated, he or she might be particularly 'windy'. This can be due to simply eating a lot of wind-inducing foods such as cabbage, beans or dried fruit, but it can also be a sign that the gut is stagnant, lacking in beneficial bacteria, housing harmful micro-organisms, or may be intolerant to a food (see Allergy, pages 98–9). Replenishing the bacteria with natural yoghurt and avoiding trigger foods can be helpful. However, if a child is painfully or excessively constipated, the cause should be investigated with a doctor or other health professional.

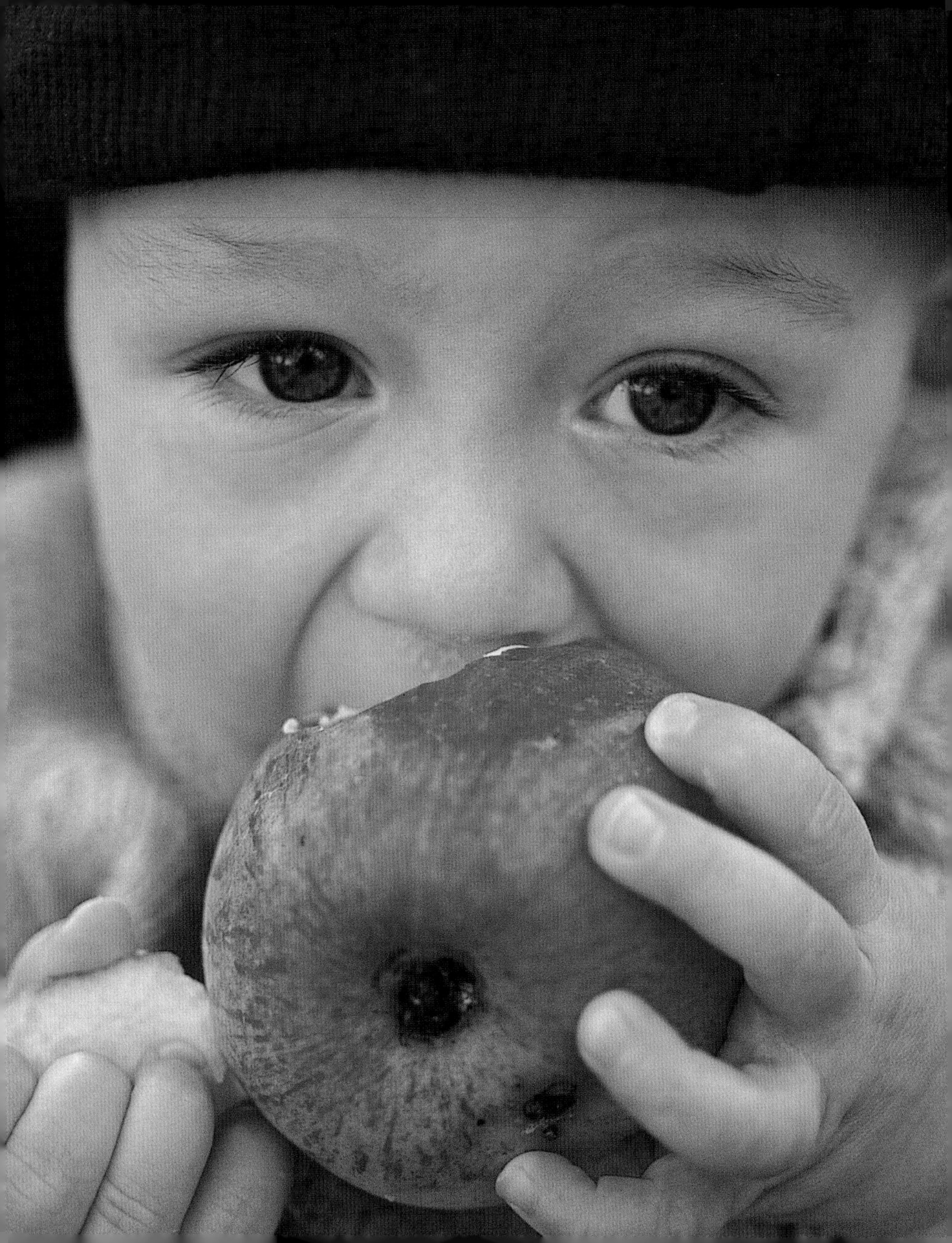

apple

If the closest your children get to apples is bobbing for them at a summer fair or toffee apples, it's certainly worth introducing them to your fruit bowl. Like most sayings, "an apple a day keeps the doctor away" is now grounded firmly in science. Apples are a wonderful source of two types of fibre: insoluble, which works like roughage, and soluble pectin (found mainly in the skin), which softens the stool by drawing water into it and bulking it out. Conversely, pectin also firms up loose stools, so it's useful for treating diarrhoea. It latches on to wastes and is good fuel for the healthy gut bacteria. Apples also contain a flavonoid called quercetin, which helps reduce inflammation and allergic reactions. The fruit's sweetness comes largely from fructose, which alongside the fibre, makes for a good gradual release of energy for children. If a child finds eating a whole apple 'boring', try adding chopped apple to a salad or cereal, or offer cooked apple for a change. And look for unusual, tasty varieties at farmers' markets rather than buy bland, imported apples. Ideally, you want this staple to be a child's favourite.

baked pork with apples

YOU COULD ROAST A LOIN, SHOULDER OR LEG OF PORK WITH THE SAME APPLE MIXTURE IN THE BOTTOM OF THE PAN, THOUGH CHOPS GO DOWN WELL WITH MOST CHILDREN.

6–8 dried ***shiitake mushrooms***
1 mugful of boiling water
2 medium crisp eating ***apples****, such as Cox's*
1/4 fennel bulb, finely sliced
4 pork chops, about 175g each
freshly ground black pepper
2 ***thyme*** *sprigs, leaves stripped*
2 ***garlic*** *cloves, peeled and crushed*
juice of 1/2 ***lemon***

Preheat the oven to 180°C/Gas 4. Put the mushrooms in a mug and fill it with boiling water.

Peel, core and slice the apples. Scatter the fennel and apples in the bottom of a roasting pan, ideally one with a lid (I use a terracotta brick). Lay the pork chops on top and season with pepper.

Drain the mushrooms and chop them into small pieces, reserving the water. Pour this over the apples and fennel.

Sprinkle the thyme leaves, garlic and lemon juice over the chops and scatter the mushroom pieces around them. Cover the dish with the lid or foil and bake for about 40 minutes, depending on the thickness of the chops. Serve with Squish squash (page 32) and steamed broccoli.

griddled apple rings

THIS IS A VERY QUICK AND DELICIOUS DESSERT THAT DOESN'T REQUIRE MUCH EFFORT. A DOLLOP OF FLAVOURED YOGHURT IS THE IDEAL COMPLEMENT, THOUGH YOU COULD, MORE INDULGENTLY, SERVE THE APPLES WITH VANILLA ICE CREAM.

3 crisp eating ***apples****, such as Cox's*
1 tbsp ***sesame seeds***
2 tsp unsalted butter
2 tsp runny ***honey***
TO SERVE
3 tbsp natural ***yoghurt***
1 tsp vanilla extract
pinch of ground ***cinnamon***

Peel, core and cut the apples into slices, about 5mm thick – rings look nice, but any shape will do.

Scatter the sesame seeds in a griddle or frying pan and toast over a high heat, shaking the pan, for about 4–5 minutes.

Add the butter and when it has melted, lay the apple rings in the pan. Drizzle over the honey. Fry the apples, turning them a couple of times, until they are golden brown and fairly soft.

In the meantime, mix the yoghurt, vanilla extract and cinnamon together in a bowl.

Put the apples on plates and drizzle with the sauce from the pan. Serve each portion topped with a dollop of flavoured yoghurt.

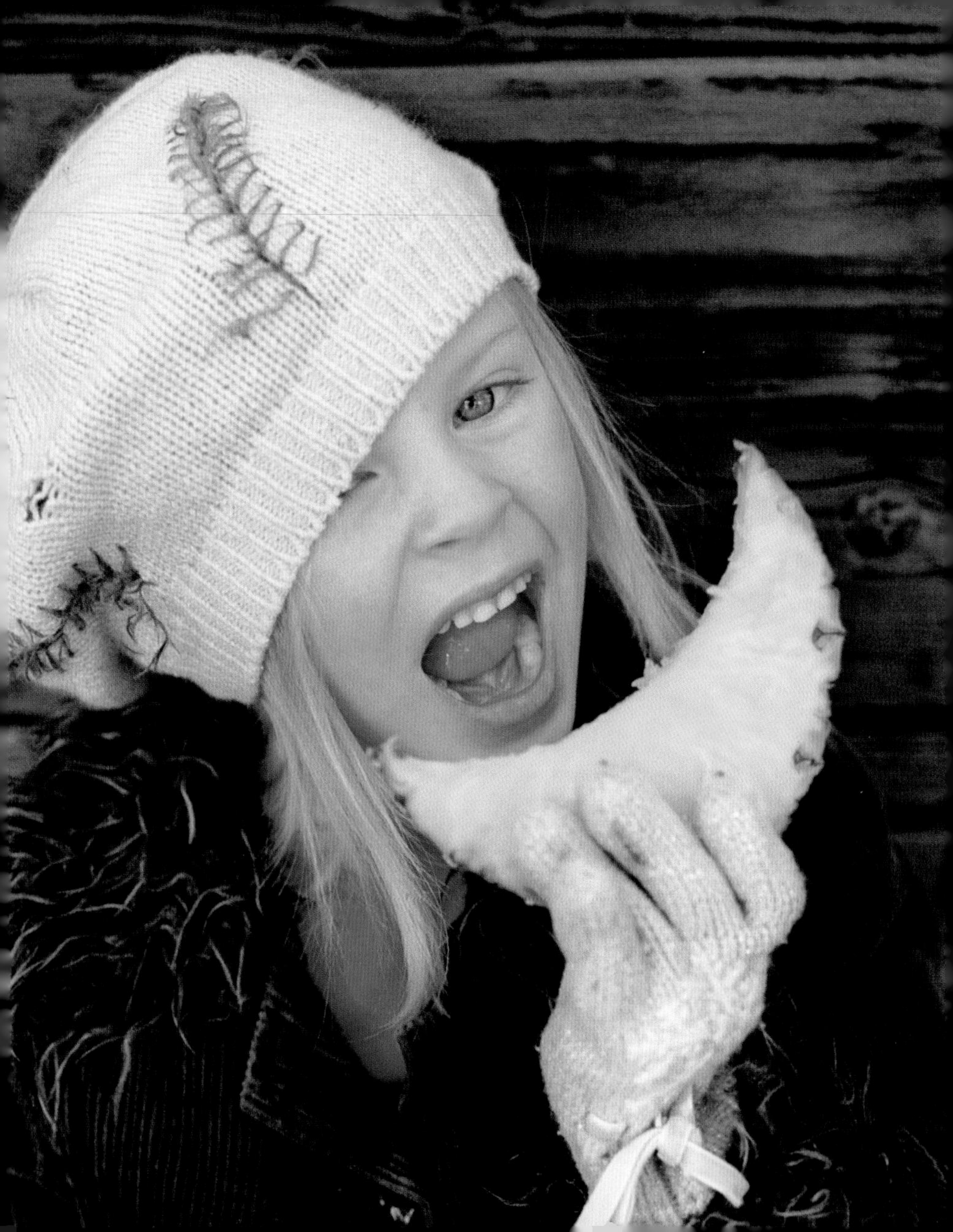

pineapple

The luscious flavour and juiciness of this tropical fruit go down well with most children and these qualities are easily matched by exceptional health benefits. Fresh pineapple is rich in a substance called bromelain, which is a sulphur-based protein-digesting enzyme. It not only helps digestion by breaking down protein, but also can help reduce inflammation in a range of conditions in children including sinusitis, sore throats and swollen joints. It's the powerful protein-digesting powers that make pineapple a popular accompaniment to meat. Bromelain is even extracted from pineapples for tablets to help digestion and lower inflammation. Pineapple is an abundant source of the mineral manganese that is essential for enzymes involved in energy production and antioxidant defence. Compounds in pineapple, known as CCS and CCZ, have been found to boost immunity and even block the growth of different types of tumour cells. Pineapple can be eaten in sweet and savoury dishes, not to mention alone. Offer your children chopped fresh pineapple as a dessert or pack into lunchboxes as a treat.

pineapple boats

THESE MAKE A FANCY LUNCH FOR CHILDREN, OR YOU COULD SERVE THEM AS A STARTER FOR A BIGGER MEAL.

2 small, ripe ***pineapples***
1 ***avocado***
200g prawns, shelled, deveined and cooked
2 tbsp natural ***yoghurt***
juice of 1/2 ***lemon***
dash of Worcestershire sauce, to taste
4–5 ***coriander*** *sprigs, roughly chopped*

Cut the pineapples in half lengthways, then cut out and discard the core. Scoop out the flesh, leaving the shells intact.

Chop half of the pineapple flesh into small pieces and put into a large bowl; save the rest for eating another time (or for the kebabs, opposite).

Halve, stone and peel the avocado, then dice the flesh. Add to the chopped pineapple with the prawns, yoghurt, lemon juice, Worcestershire sauce and coriander and toss to mix.

Just before serving, pile the prawn mix into the pineapple shells.

tropical kebabs

YOU CAN USE ANY FRUIT YOU LIKE ON THESE SKEWERS, AND EAT THEM EITHER HOT OR COLD.

- ½ *fresh* ***pineapple****, peeled and cored*
- ½ ***papaya****, peeled and deseeded*
- 2 ***kiwi fruit****, peeled*
- 1 *large* ***banana****, peeled*
- 8 *large red seedless* ***grapes***
- 4 *thin lemongrass stalks or wooden skewers*

Cut the pineapple, papaya and kiwi fruit into cubes. Slice the banana into 2cm thick rounds. Thread all the fruit on to the lemongrass sticks or skewers, alternating them (young children could do this with help).

To serve warm, preheat the grill (to high) or a barbecue. Cook the kebabs for about 5 minutes, turning occasionally to colour on all sides.

The kebabs are great on their own or they can be dipped into natural yoghurt flavoured with a little ground cinnamon and honey.

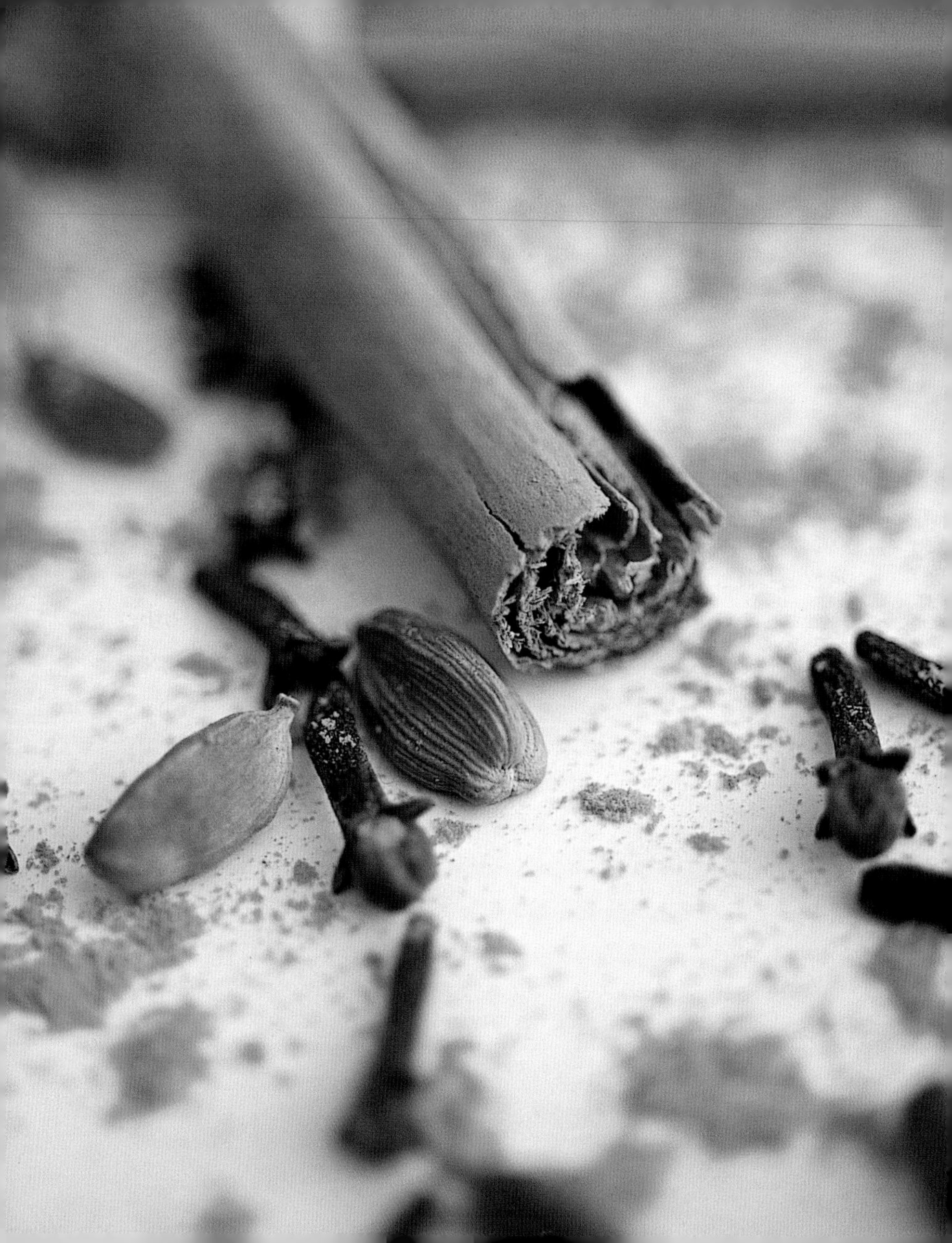

spices

One of my most vivid childhood flavour memories is of Iranian nougat studded with pistachios and scented with cardamom. It is now recognised that the wider a variety of tastes children are exposed to at a young age, the less fussy they are. Spices, used sparingly, not only transform any number of dishes, but are laden with health qualities too. Cardamom and other spices such as cinnamon, turmeric and cloves are traditional remedies for 'tummy ache'; they help to soothe gripey pains, eliminate wind and relieve nausea. Cloves and cinnamon are, in addition to digestive aids, used in traditional cold and cough remedies because of their antiviral, antibacterial and antifungal properties. Turmeric has been used for centuries in Ayurvedic medicine and now scientists are investigating its benefits in cystic fibrosis, inflammatory bowel diseases, inflammation with asthma and eczema, joint injuries and minor tummy troubles. You can make children a tasty, hot drink simply by boiling up these spices (replacing turmeric with ginger) in some water, sweetening it with honey and adding a little milk or soya milk.

dusted drumsticks

THESE ARE PRETTY SPEEDY TO PREPARE, WITH VERY TASTY RESULTS. YOU COULD ALWAYS MAKE EXTRA FOR PACKED LUNCHES.

8 ***chicken*** *drumsticks, washed and dried*
1/2 tsp ground ***cinnamon***
1/2 tsp sweet paprika
1/2 tsp smoked paprika
1/2 tsp ground ***turmeric***
2 tsp tamari (or soy sauce)
1/2 mugful of water (150ml)
1cm piece fresh root ***ginger****, peeled and grated*
2 ***garlic*** *cloves, peeled and crushed*

Preheat the oven to 190°C/Gas 5. Lay the chicken drumsticks in a roasting dish. Mix the cinnamon, paprika and turmeric together in a small bowl. With dry hands, pat the dry spice mix on to the chicken skin to coat the drumsticks lightly all over. (Younger children can help with this, just remind them to wash their hands well afterwards.)

Add the tamari to the half-mugful of water, stir in the ginger and garlic, then pour the mixture around the chicken.

Bake in the oven for 40 minutes, or until you are sure the chicken is cooked through: to test insert a thin skewer into the thickest part – the juices should run clear. Serve with brown rice and Sesame beans (page 137).

juicy fruits

THIS SUPER, EASY COMPOTE IS A POPULAR DESSERT WITH YOUNG (AND OLDER) GUESTS AND IT CAN ALSO BE EATEN AT BREAKFAST. USE ANY DRIED FRUITS YOU FANCY AND CONSIDER MAKING DOUBLE TO HAVE A SUPPLY IN THE FRIDGE FOR THE FOLLOWING DAY.

100g dried ***peaches*** *(or* ***apricots****)*
100g dried ***apple*** *rings*
50g ***raisins***
200ml water
100ml ***apple*** *juice*
10 ***cardamom*** *pods*
10 ***cloves***
2 star anise

Put all the ingredients into a saucepan and slowly bring the liquid to a simmer.

Cover the pan and leave it all to simmer over a very low heat for about 40 minutes – to allow time for the spices to infuse. (Less time will do if you're rushed.) Remove the lid if you want to make the liquor thicker but be careful not to let it boil dry. Take out the spices before serving.

This compote is delicious with natural yoghurt or, for a treat, serve it with vanilla ice cream.

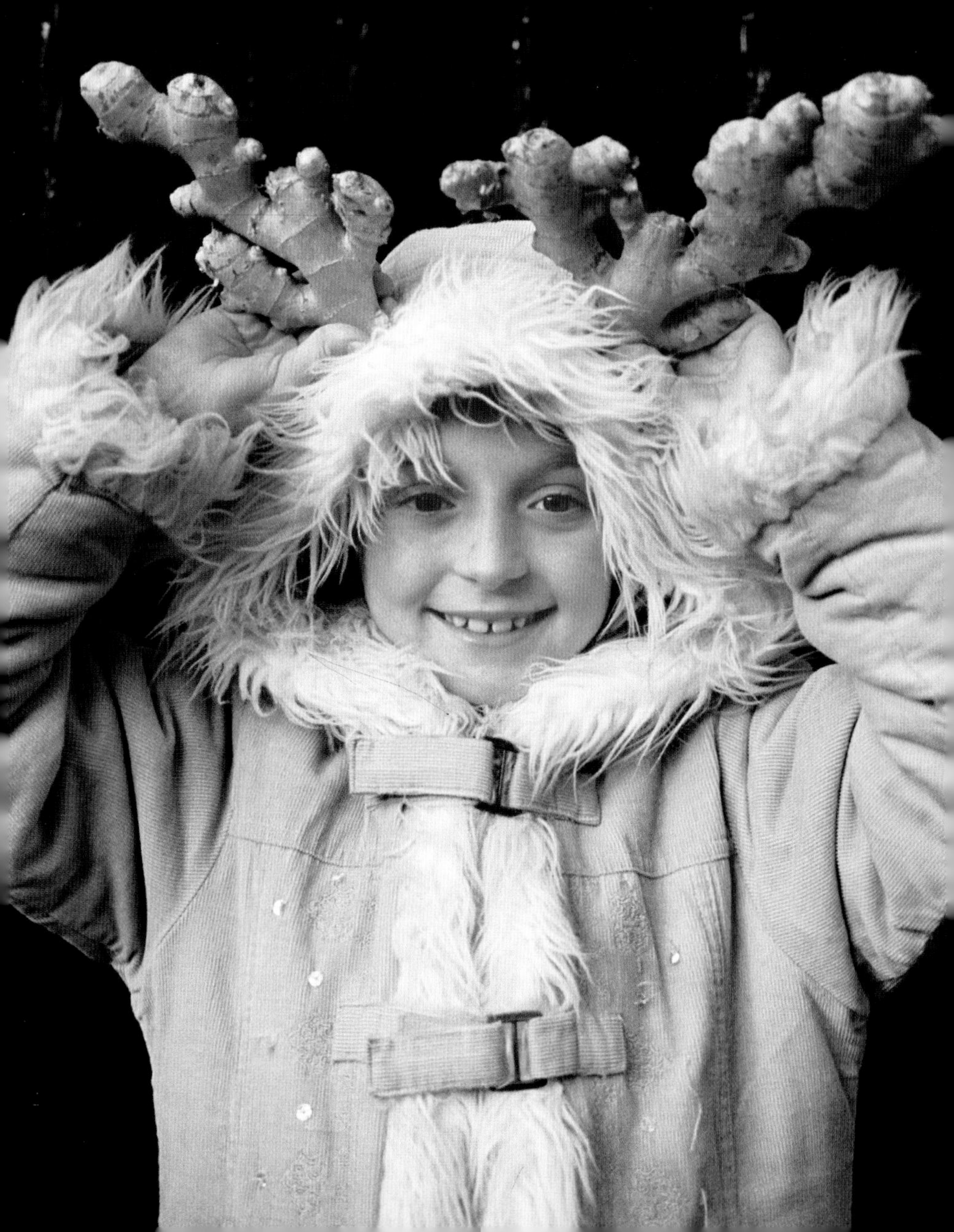

ginger

Although gingerbread men and ginger biscuits do contain ginger, it's worth incorporating this aromatic, spicy root into more foods, given its appealing taste, culinary versatility and health properties. Ginger has been used in India and China for thousands of years to treat digestive distress. It helps to expel wind and calm painful spasms, so it's useful for those things that can cause 'tummy ache'. It has been shown in scientific studies to reduce nausea, whether linked to illness or travel sickness. Herbalists also recommend ginger in the treatment of colds and coughs, partly for its warming properties, which promote useful sweating, but also because it can help calm the actual coughing. Ginger also has anti-inflammatory properties that are useful in childhood conditions such as eczema, asthma and rheumatoid arthritis. Add fresh ginger root to stews and soups, cook rice with it, or infuse in hot water and flavour with honey and lemon to make a soothing drink for a child with a cold or cough. Otherwise, left to cool, a ginger infusion makes a great base for a refreshing drink, mixed with fruit juice.

fresh fruit & ginger soup

YOU CAN SERVE THIS WARM OR COLD, DEPENDING ON YOUR TASTE AND THE SEASON. USE ANY FRUITS YOU HAVE TO HAND.

2 ripe ***peaches***
8 ***strawberries****, hulled*
1 ***banana****, peeled*
250ml ***pineapple*** *juice*
2.5cm piece fresh root ***ginger****, peeled and grated*
1 tbsp ***honey***
4 heaped tsp natural ***yoghurt****, to serve*

Halve, stone and roughly chop the peaches; halve the strawberries unless they are very small; cut the banana into chunky slices.

Put the pineapple juice, ginger and honey in a saucepan, bring to the boil and boil for a minute, then turn down the heat to a simmer. Add the fruit and simmer gently for 3–4 minutes, then take off the heat.

Serve the 'soup' while it's still warm, or leave it to cool and eat it later. Either way, top each portion with a dollop of natural yoghurt.

fish in sleeping bags

OPENING UP THE 'SLEEPING BAGS' ON YOUR PLATE IS PART OF THE FUN OF THIS DISH. IT GOES WELL WITH SESAME BEANS (PAGE 137) AND PLAIN BROWN RICE. GET YOUR CHILDREN TO HELP YOU MAKE AND FILL THE SLEEPING BAGS.

4 ***fish*** *fillets, such as haddock or snapper*
2 ***garlic*** *cloves, peeled and crushed*
2.5cm piece fresh root ***ginger****, peeled and grated*
1 ***lime****, halved*
2 tsp ***sesame*** *oil*
1 small can ***coconut*** *milk*

Preheat the oven to 180°C/Gas 4. Cut four pieces of greaseproof paper and fold each in half – folded, they need to be big enough to fold up over the fish and scrunch up to seal.

Lay a fish fillet in the middle of each double sheet and scatter the garlic and ginger over and under the fish. Squeeze a little lime juice and drizzle some sesame oil on top of each fillet. Fold up the sides of the paper, then spoon about 2 tbsp coconut milk on to each fish fillet.

Bring the edges of the paper to meet over the fish and roll and scrunch them together to form a little 'sleeping bag'. Place the 'bags' on a baking tray and bake in the oven for about 15 minutes, depending on the thickness of the fillets.

Serve the fish in their sleeping bags on plates for children to open themselves – making sure they do so carefully to avoid escaping steam.

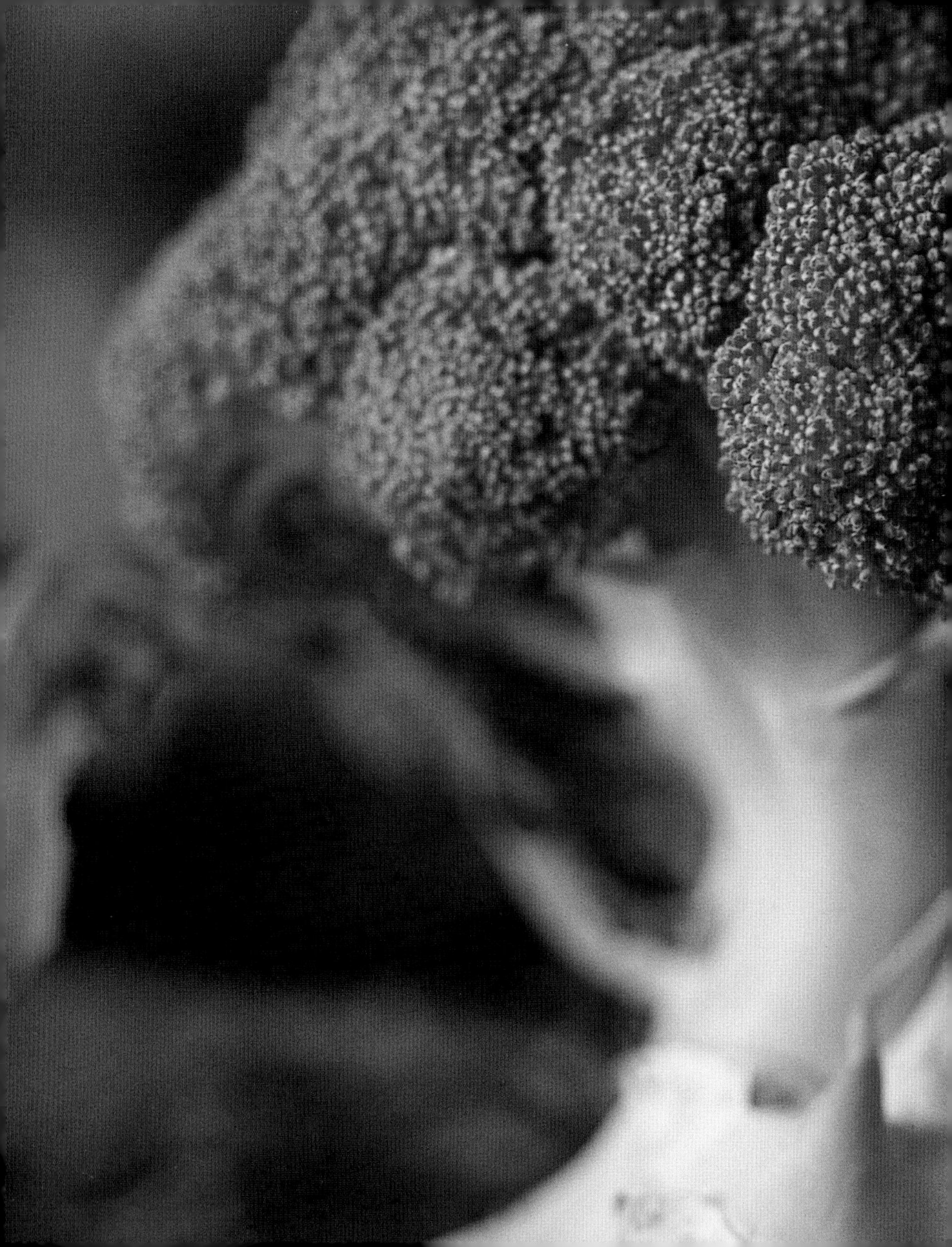

broccoli

A member of the brassica family, broccoli is generally more popular with children than its cousins – Brussels sprouts, kale cauliflower and cabbage – and it is loaded with goodness. Including this extraordinarily nutritious vegetable in your child's diet from an early age is the best way to ensure he or she develops a taste for it. Broccoli contains a good dose of fibre that keeps the bowels moving and feeds the beneficial bacteria there, which help keep tummy bugs and other problems at bay. It is also loaded with calcium, which is useful for healthy bones, particularly for any child who does not tolerate milk. A group of sulphur-containing chemicals called glucosinolates in broccoli (and other brassicas) are important for a healthy liver and some have even shown anti-cancer properties. One glucosinolate, indole-3-carbinol, is needed to process oestrogen, so as girls reach puberty it helps balance their menstrual cycles. Broccoli and kale are loaded with other antioxidants such as vitamin C and beta carotene, important for immunity, skin, lungs, eyes and much more.

garlicky broccoli stir-fry

MANY CHILDREN WILL LOVE ANYTHING THAT TASTES OF SLIGHTLY OILY GARLIC, EVEN IF IT'S GREEN VEG! I REMEMBER 'LOVING' SNAILS ON A TRIP TO BRUSSELS AS A CHILD WHEN REALLY IT WAS JUST MOPPING UP THE GARLIC BUTTER THAT DID IT. YOU CAN, OF COURSE, ADD ANY OTHER VEG TO THIS STIR-FRY SIDE DISH.

1 large head of ***broccoli****, trimmed*
1 tbsp olive oil
1 tsp Chinese five spice powder (optional)
3 ***garlic*** *cloves, peeled and crushed*
1 tbsp tamari (or soy sauce)
2 tbsp water

Break the broccoli into small florets and roughly chop the stalks.

In a wok or large frying pan, heat the olive oil, together with the five spice powder if using, for a minute. Add the broccoli, garlic, tamari and water. Stir-fry for 4–5 minutes until the broccoli is cooked through but still slightly crunchy.

Serve straight away with brown rice and any main dish, such as Chickpea & coconut curry (page 90) or Sticky chicken (page 153).

spotty mash

THIS IS A CUNNING WAY TO 'HIDE' GREEN VEG, ALTHOUGH THE BROCCOLI DOESN'T REALLY DISGUISE ITSELF AT ALL! SERVE WITH ANY FISH, CHICKEN OR MEAT DISH, PERHAPS EASY ROAST LAMB (PAGE 129). YOU COULD FRY UP LEFTOVERS WITH EGGS TO MAKE 'BUBBLE & SQUEAK' FOR BREAKFAST THE NEXT DAY.

3 medium ***sweet potatoes****,*
peeled and diced
1 large head of ***broccoli****,*
stalks removed
knob of butter
100ml milk or ***soya*** *milk*
2 tbsp Parmesan cheese,
freshly grated

Boil the sweet potatoes in a large saucepan for about 15 minutes until they are quite soft. Meanwhile, roughly chop the broccoli florets. Add them to the pan and simmer for another 5 minutes until they, too, are quite soft (more so than if you were going to eat the broccoli as a side veg).

Drain the vegetables and put them back in the pan. Squish them with a potato masher, adding the butter, milk and Parmesan as you do so. (Young children can do this.) Serve at once.

NOTE It's best to leave out the broccoli stalks here – eat them with the Chickpea dip (page 89.)

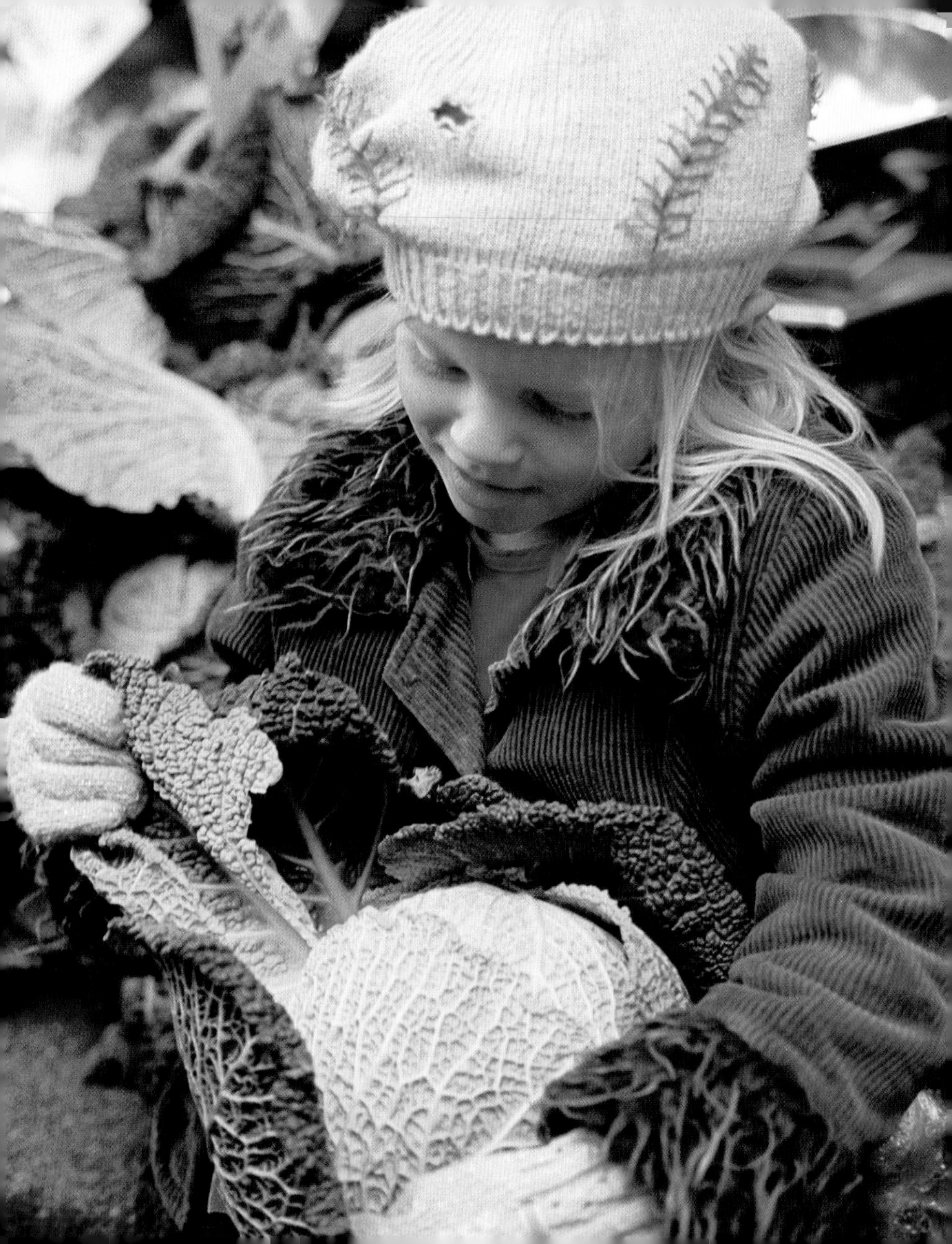

cabbage

Many of us off were turned of this 'wonderveg' as children by soggy school dinner cabbage and the sulphurous smell let off during overcooking. Even with fewer children eating canteen meals, it remains well off the list of favourites. Cooking cabbage in cunning ways is the way to slot its goodness into your child's diet. The fibre and sulphur in cabbage give it its windy, smelly reputation, but these two elements also bestow wonderful health benefits. The fibre helps prevent constipation, feeds good bacteria and helps makes sure wastes are cleared out of the body efficiently. Sulphur is not only important for the liver to work well, but is also needed for healthy skin, particularly in childhood conditions such as eczema. Like broccoli, cabbage is useful for helping to balance girls' menstrual cycles by optimising the way the liver processes oestrogen. The high levels of vitamin C in cabbage are used in the liver, as well as for boosting the immune system and skin health. To brighten up a meal, so it appeals more to children, use red cabbage or Savoy with its crinkly textured leaves... and don't overcook it!

cabbage & bacon

OF THE DISHES PREPARED BY MY MOTHER WHEN I WAS A CHILD, THIS IS ONE OF MY FAVOURITES. I'VE ADDED IN THE FENNEL SEEDS AND PARSLEY BUT YOU CAN EASILY LEAVE OUT EITHER OR BOTH IF YOUR CHILDREN DON'T LIKE THEM.

120g smoked back bacon, derinded and chopped
1 tbsp olive oil
1½ tsp fennel seeds
freshly ground black pepper
½ Savoy ***cabbage****, cored and shredded*
5 tbsp water
2 tbsp chopped ***parsley***

Place a large saucepan over a medium heat, add the bacon, olive oil and fennel seeds and stir them for 3 or 4 minutes, seasoning with a little pepper.

Tip in the cabbage, add the water and mix it all together. Cover and cook over a low heat for about 10 minutes until the cabbage is tender. Stir in the chopped parsley.

Serve at once, as a side dish. It goes really well with Baked turkey rolls (page 152).

leaf rolls

ROLLING YOUR OWN FOOD AND DIPPING IT IN SAUCE MAKES IT ALL MUCH MORE FUN. THIS IS INSPIRED BY MY DELIGHT AS A CHILD OF SHARING DUCK PANCAKES AT A BIG TABLE IN A CHINESE RESTAURANT WITH A SPINNING MIDDLE. YOU COULD HAVE SHREDDED CHICKEN OR SLICED SMOKED TOFU INSTEAD OF THE SALMON.

4 small ***salmon*** *steaks*
1 ***carrot****, peeled*
½ ***cucumber***
large handful of ***bean sprouts***
12 large Savoy ***cabbage*** *leaves (at least)*

FOR THE DIPPING SAUCE
6 tbsp tamari (or soy sauce)
3 tbsp toasted ***sesame*** *oil*
2 tbsp sweet chilli sauce

Steam, poach or bake the salmon steaks until just tender, then tip into a serving bowl and roughly break them up with a fork, checking for any small bones as you do so.

Finely slice the carrot lengthways and cut the cucumber into strips. Arrange on serving plates with the bean sprouts.

Mix the tamari, sesame oil and sweet chilli sauce in a couple of small serving bowls or individual soy sauce dipping bowls.

Bring a large saucepan of water to the boil and blanch the cabbage leaves for about 3 minutes. Rinse, pat dry and lay them on a warm plate.

Get the children to roll some salmon and vegetables in a cabbage leaf and dip it into the sauce before eating each mouthful.

NOTE After blanching, the cabbage leaves can be kept warm in a steamer over gently simmering water and taken out as required.

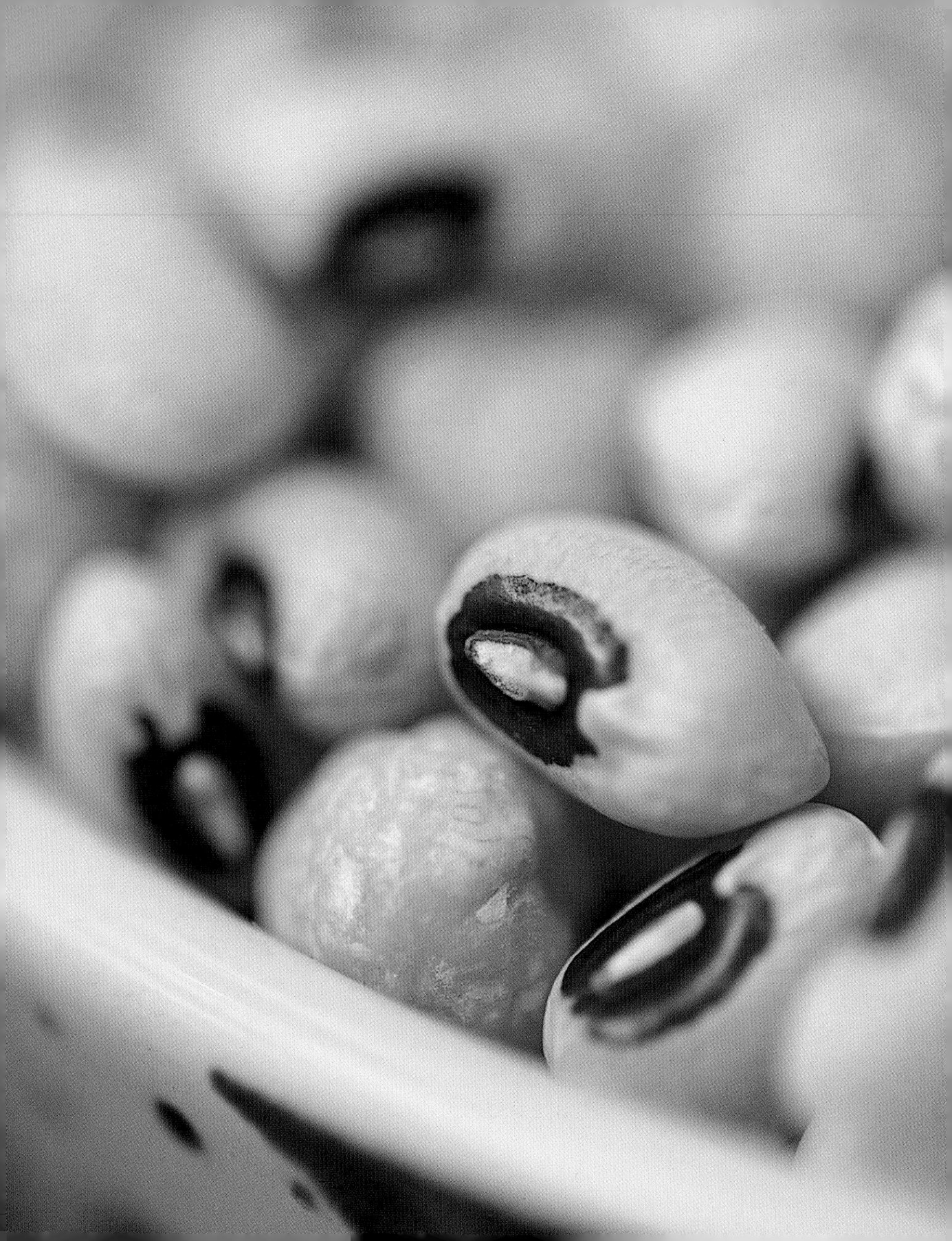

dried beans & chickpeas

"Beans beans, good for your heart. The more you eat, the more you ...." an age-old verse that rings true, although I imagine the first line was coined simply to rhyme rather than because the 'poet' knew it was a medical fact! Beans and chickpeas are, indeed, very likely to cause wind because of all the fibre in them. They contain the insoluble variety, which helps increase the bulk of the stool and prevent constipation, also reducing the risk of digestive disorders like irritable bowel syndrome. But fibre doesn't just keep your children regular. The soluble fibre in beans makes a gel-like substance in the gut that slows down the release of blood sugar after a meal, to provide longer-term energy rather than the quick burst obtained from low-fibre foods. This is particularly beneficial for hyperactive children. Darker beans, such as black and kidney beans, are good sources of manganese, folic acid and iron, and their skins contains protective antioxidants. All pulses contain high levels of the mineral molybdenum, which is essential for the body to handle the sulphites found in many processed foods.

bean & bacon soup

THE SALTINESS OF THE BACON GOES WONDERFULLY WITH THE SWEETNESS OF THE BEANS IN THIS SOUP. USE ANY BEANS YOU FANCY AND, AS ALWAYS, BEST TO COOK THEM FROM DRIED... THOUGH I FIND I NEVER GET ROUND TO IT!

250g smoked bacon or gammon, fat removed
1 tbsp olive oil
1 large ***onion****, peeled and finely diced*
2 ***celery*** *sticks, sliced*
2 x 400g cans borlotti, haricot or butter ***beans*** *(in water rather than brine), drained and rinsed*
freshly ground black pepper
1 litre vegetable stock
handful of ***parsley****, chopped*

Cut the bacon into 1cm cubes and cook in a large saucepan (without oil) until tender. Remove half of it and keep aside.

Add the olive oil to the pan, then the onion and celery and cook, stirring, over a low heat until the onion is soft. Tip the beans into the pan, season with a little pepper and pour in the stock. Bring to a simmer and simmer, covered, for about 30 minutes. Meanwhile, chop the reserved bacon into smaller pieces.

When the soup is ready, add the parsley and then whiz, using a hand-held stick blender until you have a thick, warming soup. Stir in the bacon pieces and serve.

NOTE If you want to make the soup a bit less thick, just add another 200ml water.

chickpea dip

THIS IS A VARIATION ON A THEME OF TRADITIONAL HOUMMOUS. EVEN YOUNGER CHILDREN CAN HELP – BY DROPPING THE INGREDIENTS INTO THE BLENDER.

400g can ***chickpeas*** *(in water rather than brine), drained and rinsed*
juice of 1 ***lemon***
*2 tbsp tahini (****sesame seed*** *paste)*
1 ***garlic*** *clove, peeled*
4–6 ***basil*** *leaves*
4–6 ***mint*** *leaves*
2 heaped tbsp natural ***yoghurt***
good pinch of sea salt
4 tbsp olive oil

Put all the ingredients, except the olive oil, in a food processor or free-standing blender. Whiz them together until smooth, gradually pouring in the olive oil through the feeder funnel. If necessary (and still with the motor running), add a little cold water until you get the consistency you want.

Serve the dip with hot brown pitta bread and vegetable sticks, or with Avocado dip & chips (page 178) if you like.

chickpea & coconut curry

YOU CAN, OF COURSE, COOK DRIED CHICKPEAS FOR THIS CURRY, INSTEAD OF USING CANNED ONES AS I DO.

1 heaped tsp ground cumin seeds
1 tsp ground coriander
½ tsp ground ***turmeric***
2 tbsp grated dried ***coconut***
1 ***onion****, peeled and finely sliced*
1cm piece fresh root ***ginger****, peeled and grated*
2 ***garlic*** *cloves, peeled and crushed*
400ml can ***coconut*** *milk*
400g can ***tomatoes***
2 x 400g cans ***chickpeas*** *(in water rather than brine), drained and rinsed*
good pinch of sea salt

Put the cumin, coriander, turmeric and dried coconut in a large, dry saucepan over a medium heat and stir for a minute or two until the coconut is slightly browned.

Add the onion, ginger and garlic with 3 tbsp of the coconut milk and stir over a low heat for about 10 minutes, adding a little water to avoid sticking.

Then add the tomatoes and chickpeas with the rest of the coconut milk and a good pinch of salt. Stir, then cover and leave to simmer for about 30 minutes, stirring occasionally. Add a little water if you want more sauce.

Serve the curry with brown rice and steamed green veg, such as broccoli or spinach.

lamb & bean hotpot

THIS IS A WONDERFULLY WARMING, COMFORTING DISH – A SORT OF LANCASHIRE HOTPOT-CASSOULET HYBRID!

1 tbsp olive oil
8 small or 4 large ***lamb*** *chops*
1 large ***onion****, peeled and finely diced*
2 ***garlic*** *cloves, peeled and crushed*
2 ***thyme*** *sprigs (or 1 tsp dried thyme)*
2 ***rosemary*** *sprigs*
dash of Worcestershire sauce, to taste
400g can chopped ***tomatoes***
1 bay leaf
400g can haricot ***beans*** *(in water rather than brine), drained and rinsed*
300ml boiling water

Preheat the oven to 180°C/Gas 4. Heat the olive oil in a large frying pan and brown the chops on each side, then transfer them to an ovenproof casserole dish and set aside.

Add the onion, garlic, thyme, rosemary, Worcestershire sauce, tomatoes and bay leaf to the frying pan and cook, stirring, over a low heat for about 10 minutes. Tip the beans into the pan, stir in the hot water and warm through.

Spoon this mixture over the lamb chops. Put on the lid or cover the dish with foil and cook in the oven for 50 minutes.

Serve the hotpot with Veggie rosti (page 162) or steamed green veg.

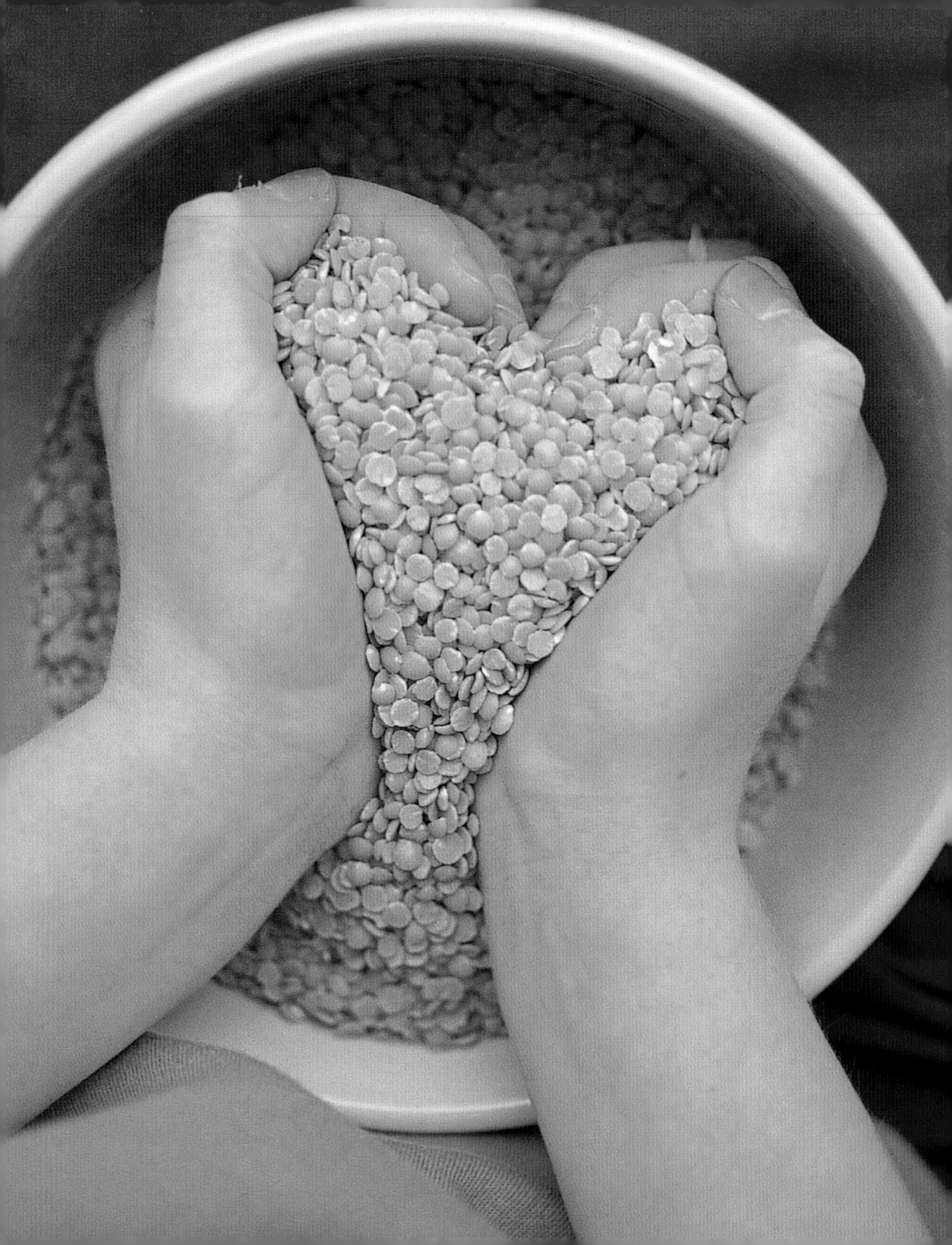

lentils

Lentils, the ‘poor man’s meat’, crop up in many ancient cultures. In Jewish tradition, they were served to mourners, their round shape representing the life cycle, with no beginning and no end. Ancient Egyptians thought they enlightened the mind. Whatever your beliefs, lentils are an inexpensive staple that provides a richness of protein, fibre and other nutrients. After soya beans, they have the highest protein content in the vegetable kingdom, so they make a nourishing meal, especially for vegetarian children. Although lentils are packed with fibre (and can be ‘windy’), they are more digestible than most beans and chickpeas and don’t need soaking before cooking. The fibre they contain will help keep the guts moving. Even if your child doesn’t suffer from constipation, ensuring the bowels are eliminated effectively is important not just for gut health, but also for hormone balance and general detoxification. The slow-releasing fuel from high-fibre lentils is good for a gradual energy supply. Alongside this, the B vitamins they contain are great for energy, growth and calm moods in your children.

dahl

MARIA PEREIRA, FROM GOA, PREPARED THIS DISH FOR ME WHEN I WAS A CHILD AND EVER SINCE SHE TAUGHT ME HOW TO MAKE IT, IT'S BEEN A FIRM FAVOURITE – TASTY, EASY AND CHEAP TOO.

1 mugful of split orange ***lentils***
1 tsp olive oil
1 large ***onion****, peeled and chopped*
5 ***garlic*** *cloves, peeled and crushed*
1 tsp ground coriander
1 tsp ground cumin
1 tsp ground ***turmeric***
3 mugfuls of water
400g canned chopped ***tomatoes***

Wash the lentils well in a sieve and check for any little bits of grit.

Heat the olive oil in a large saucepan and soften the onion and garlic with the spices over a low heat, adding a little of the water if they seem as though they are likely to burn.

Add the lentils, the water and tomatoes and bring to the boil. Immediately cover the pan, lower the heat and leave it all to simmer for about 45 minutes, stirring regularly to make sure the mixture is not sticking at the bottom. If it starts to become too thick, add a little more water.

Eat with brown rice or baked potatoes and steamed green veg.

lentil stacks & minty sauce

THESE ARE A GREAT ALTERNATIVE TO MEAT BURGERS AND THEY GO DOWN WELL IN WHOLEMEAL PITTA POCKETS WITH SLICES OF FRESH TOMATO AND LETTUCE. THIS QUANTITY MAKES EIGHT SMALL STACKS.

1 tbsp olive oil
1 small ***onion****, peeled and finely diced*
1 tsp ground cumin
175g split red ***lentils***
600ml vegetable stock
3 tbsp fine ***oatmeal*** *(see note)*
1 ***egg****, beaten*
FOR THE SAUCE
3 tbsp natural ***yoghurt***
6–8 ***mint*** *leaves, very finely chopped*

Preheat the oven to 200°C/Gas 6. Heat the olive oil in a large saucepan and soften the onion with the cumin over a low heat for a few minutes. Stir in the lentils and the stock. Bring to the boil, then turn the heat down and simmer for 20 minutes. Leave the cooked lentils to cool a little, then stir in the oatmeal and beaten egg. Line a baking tray with greaseproof paper. Wet your hands and form the mush into eight small patties (young children can help here). Put them on the lined baking tray and bake in the oven for 10 minutes.

Meanwhile, stir the sauce ingredients together, to serve with the lentil stacks when they're ready.

NOTE If you do not have fine oatmeal, simply whiz porridge oats in a blender for a minute.

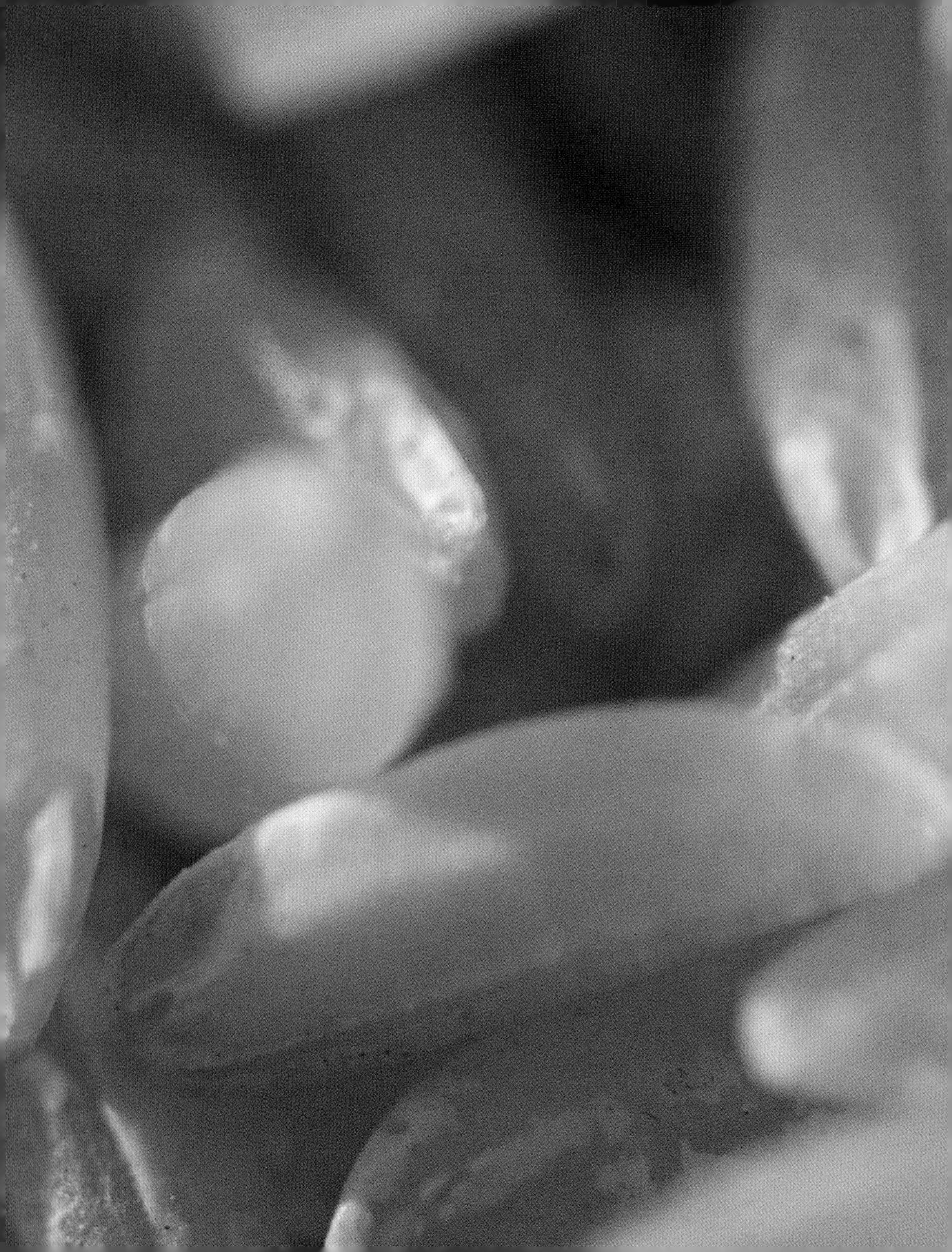

allergy

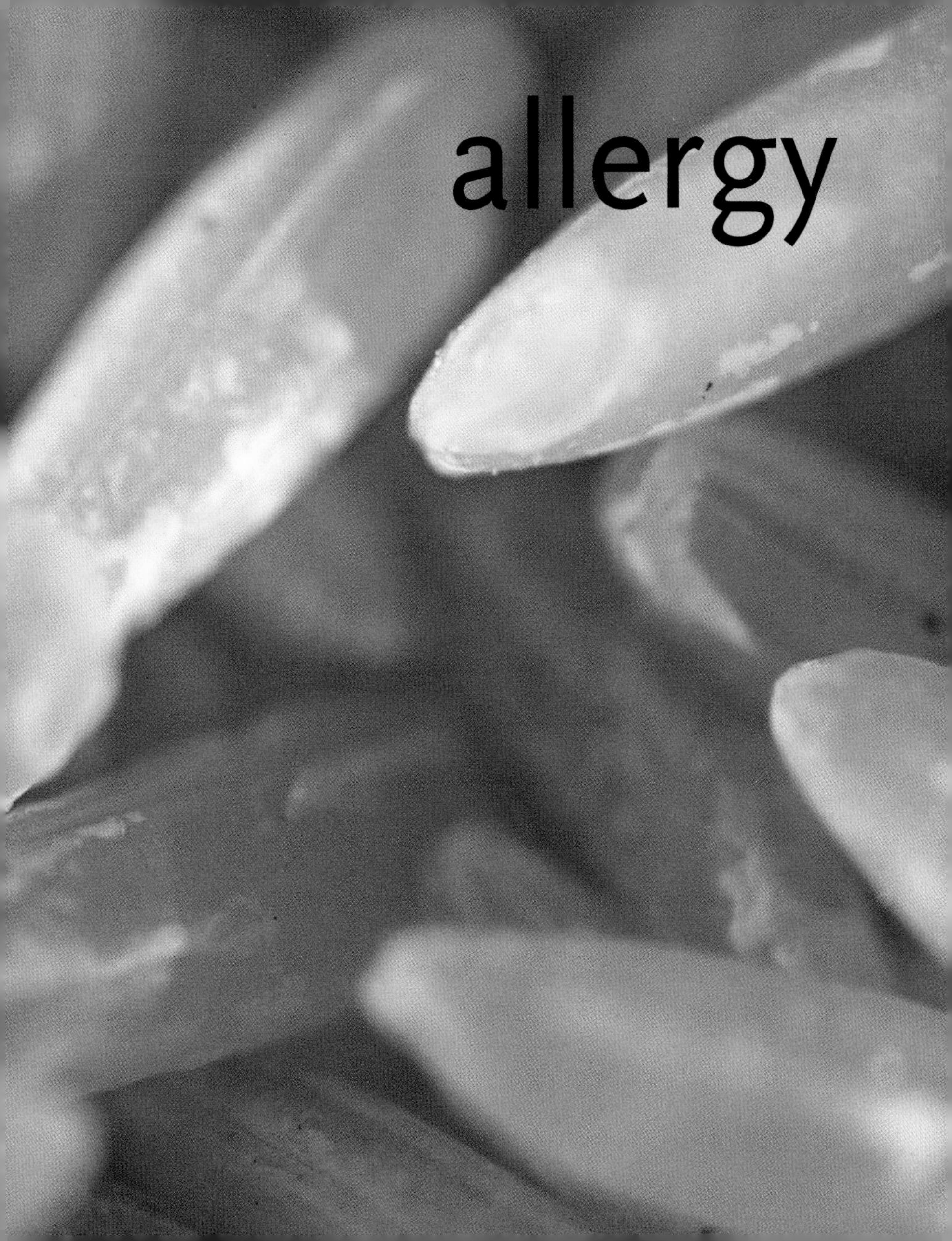

Even 15 or 20 years ago, food allergies and intolerances were a rarity – a parent hosting a child's birthday party would only occasionally have to contend with a guest who couldn't eat a particular food. Nowadays, allergies – not just to foods – are increasingly common amongst children. They are thought to affect as many as one in three but exactly why, is not clear. They are possibly due to a widespread decline in our immunity, an increased burden on our immune system, or perhaps a bit of both. Suffice to say that food sensitivities can contribute to a range of symptoms as varied as bloating, lethargy, rashes or serious reactions such as dramatic weight loss or anaphylactic shock, but much can be done to alleviate the problems.

An allergy is when the body alters its normal immune response in some way, due to the presence of an 'offending' substance, or allergen. Common allergens are dairy foods, soy, wheat, eggs and peanuts. Some people differentiate between allergy and intolerance, although often the two are used interchangeably. If there is a distinction, then food allergy usually refers to an immediate response, for example a strawberry triggers a rash straight away. Food intolerance on the other hand, usually refers to a reaction caused by a build-up from regular exposure to the allergen, so the symptoms are caused by regularly consuming an allergy-provoking food. Delayed food reactions seem to be caused by the gut's inability to prevent partially digested food from getting into the bloodstream. So dealing with food sensitivities is not just a matter of avoiding the allergens, but also looking at supporting the body's digestive capacity and immune response.

One of the most daunting issues about your child being diagnosed with a food allergy or intolerance is "What on earth do I feed him or her instead?" Another is a niggling worry that by avoiding a significant food group, (s)he may well be missing out on nutrients essential for good health and optimum growth and development. There are plenty of ways to make sure your child is getting a full spectrum of nutrients, whatever the intolerance. It's crucial, if you think your child is reacting negatively to any foods, to work with your doctor or another health professional. That way you are likely to find the triggers more easily (if they are not clear) and ensure you have good alternatives, so that you don't restrict your child's diet too much.

A traditional naturopathic diet to detect and eliminate allergies consists of lamb, rice and pears, all considered to be unlikely allergens. The wonderfoods in this chapter are typically low-allergenic, but they also provide nutrients that help gut health and immunity. All over the world traditional diets exclude certain foods, and people live long, healthy lives anyway. Think of the typical Thai cuisine, which doesn't know the meaning of milk or wheat products – how nutritious and tasty it is, and you can see that by making a few shifts in your shopping trolley, you can give your child great food.

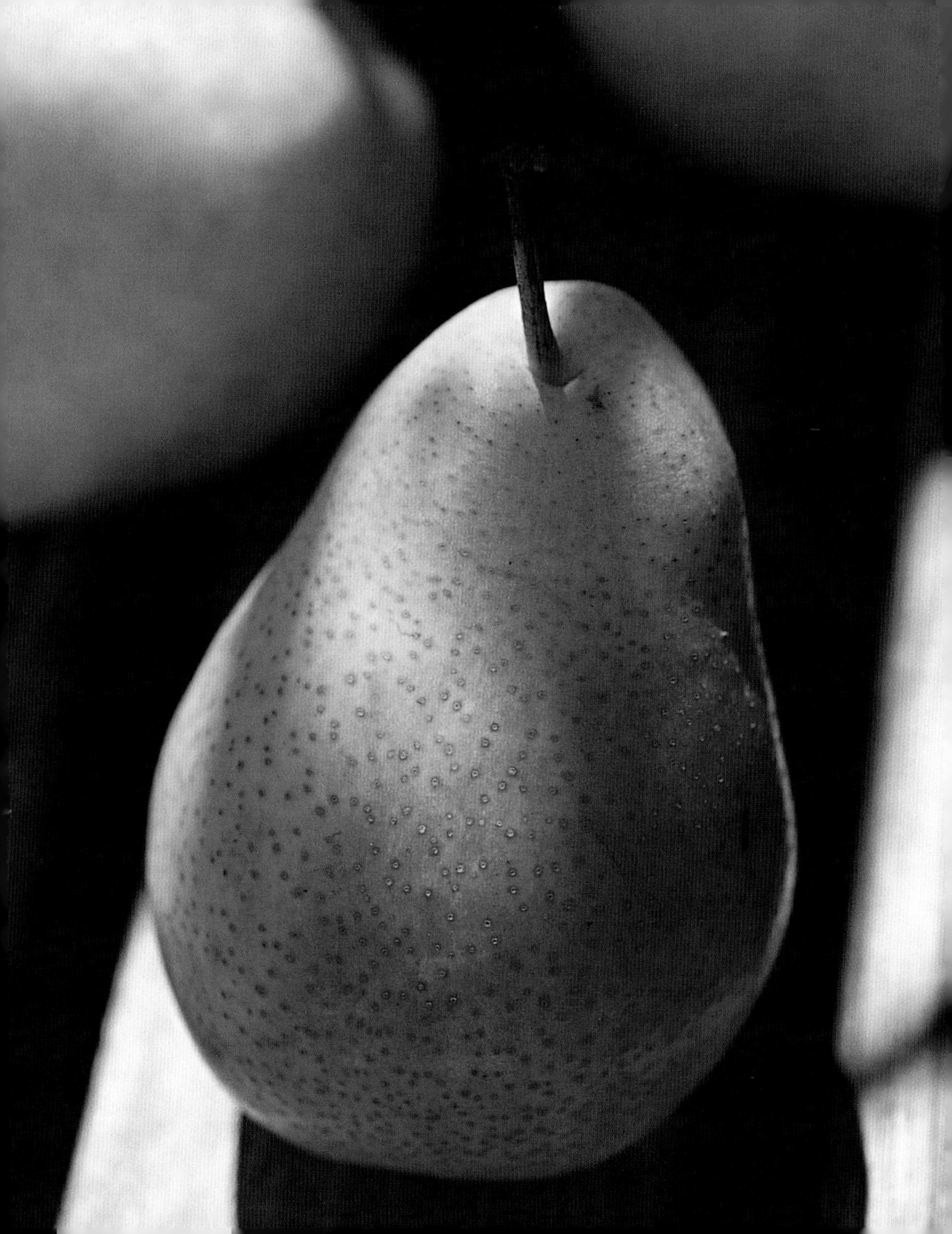

pear

Even exotic fruits struggle to beat a ripe, juicy, buttery Williams pear, which leaves juice dribbling down your child's arms and chin. Served with other fruits, dried fruits, a yoghurt or cheese, pears make a great snack, well beyond baby finger food days. Their mild flavour belies the excellent health benefits of pears, which Homer referred to as a gift from the gods. Although it is not well researched scientifically, pears are considered to be one of the least likely foods to trigger an allergic reaction. They are loaded with alkalising minerals, fibre and water, all of which are helpful for poor digestion and constipation – symptoms that often accompany food intolerances. The soluble fibre, pectin, in pears is useful for helping to ferry waste products out of the body, again useful if your child reacts with digestive symptoms to other foods. Pears, like many fruits, are a good source of the immune-boosting, skin-healing antioxidant, vitamin C, as well as the important mineral, potassium, which has many roles in the body including maintaining heartbeat, muscle contraction and the messaging between nerves.

pear & parma rolls

THESE MAKE A GREAT BASE FOR A PACKED LUNCH OR A TEATIME SNACK. USE FINELY SLICED CURED HAM, AS THIS IS EASY TO ROLL.

8 slices Parma or Serrano ham
a little cider vinegar or balsamic vinegar
2 firm, ripe ***pears***

Simply lay out the slices of cured ham on a clean surface and, using your fingers, rub a little cider vinegar on each slice.

Quarter and core the pears and lay a pear wedge at the end of each slice of Parma ham. Roll up each ham slice to enclose the pear and serve, or wrap in waxed paper or cling film to pack into lunchboxes.

baked pears

THESE MAKE A DELICATELY SWEET DESSERT THAT CAN BE SERVED WITH SOYA CREAM, NATURAL YOGHURT OR ICE CREAM. INSTEAD OF APPLE JUICE, YOU COULD USE WATER AND A SPOONFUL OF HONEY.

4 firm, ripe ***pears***
2 tbsp ***raisins***
1cm piece fresh root **ginger**, *peeled and grated*
1 ***cinnamon*** *stick*
400ml ***apple*** *juice*
2 tbsp ***sunflower seeds***

Preheat the oven to 180°C/Gas 4. Peel, halve and core the pears and lay them, cut side up, in an ovenproof dish. Scatter the raisins and ginger around them and add the cinnamon stick (small children can help here).

Pour the apple juice over the pears and bake the lot in the oven for 30 minutes.

Before serving, remove the cinnamon stick and scatter sunflower seeds over the fruit.

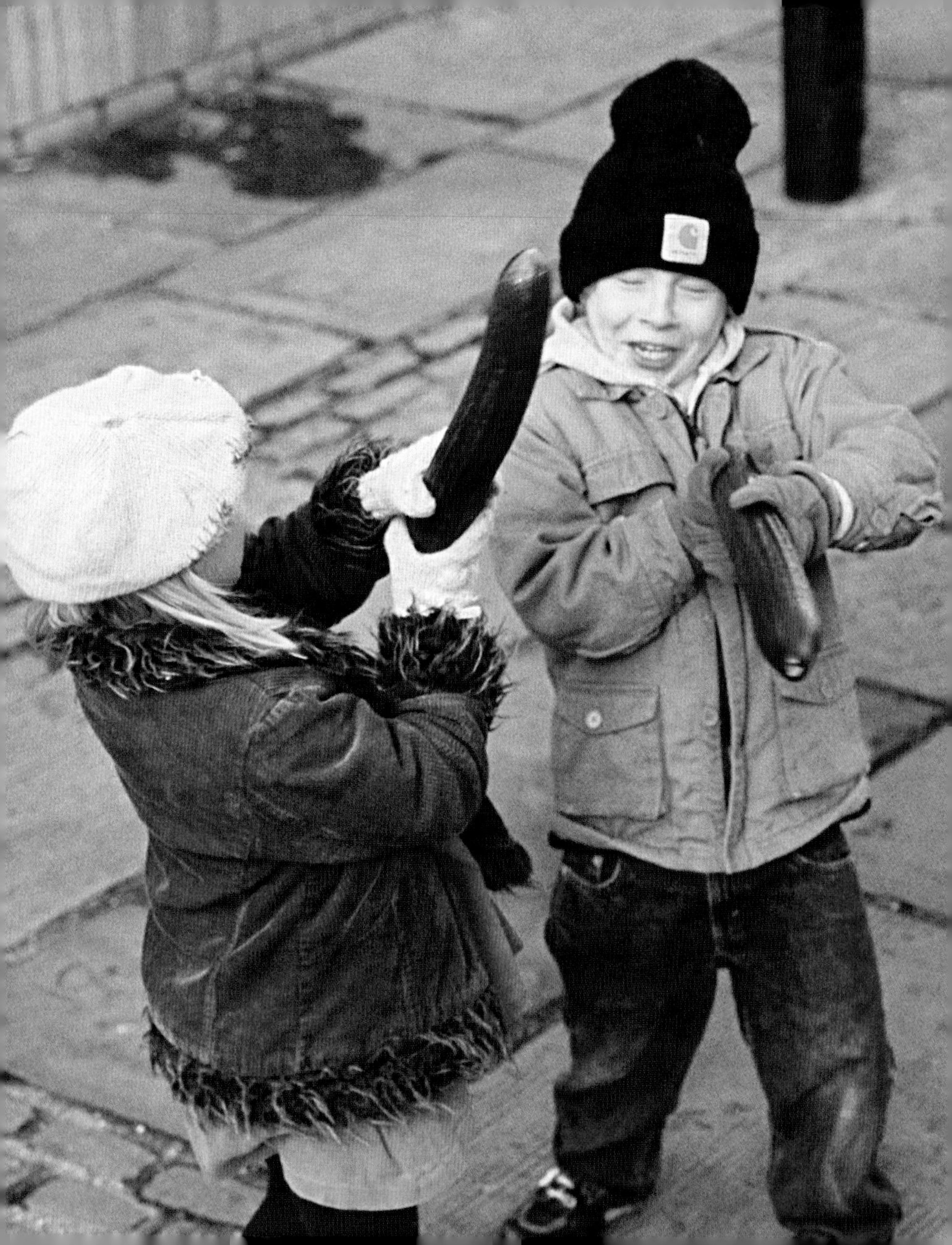

cucumber

The saying, "cool as a cucumber" is not for nothing. This salad vegetable is 95% water so it has relatively little nutritional value, but it is the juicy, hydrating properties that make it so wonderful. For centuries, before the days of fridges or vacuum flasks, cucumbers were an excellent way to 'carry' cool liquid in arid deserts. Their water and mineral content makes them cleansing and a powerful diuretic, in other words, they facilitate the passage of wastes through the kidneys. Getting your children to eat fruit and veg like cucumber is a great way to up their water intake. Cucumbers contain the mineral silica, which is important for healthy connective tissue such as cellular 'glue', muscles, tendons, ligaments and cartilage, as well as bone. The cooling nature of cucumber can be beneficial externally too, for example on your child's skin if it is mildly sunburnt. Most cucumbers sold in shops have been waxed to prevent moisture evaporation and to extend their shelf-life, so you may like to peel them. Unfortunately though, if you peel them, you lose out on much of their fibre and nutrient content.

edible spoons

THERE'S SOMETHING MUCH MORE FUN AND TASTY ABOUT EATING WITH YOUR HANDS. THIS CAN BE AN AFTERNOON SNACK OR FORM PART OF A LUNCH, PERHAPS ALONGSIDE CHICKPEA DIP (PAGE 89).

200g can ***tuna*** *in brine, drained*
110g cottage cheese or ***soya yoghurt***
juice of ½ ***lemon***
1 tbsp ***flax (linseed)*** *or* ***hemp seed*** *oil*
1 tbsp chopped ***parsley***
1 ***cucumber***

Flake the tuna into a bowl. Add the cottage cheese, lemon juice, oil and parsley and mash together, using a fork, until well blended and fairly smooth. (Young children can do this.)

Cut the cucumber into strips, at least 8cm long and 2cm thick.

Pile the tuna mash on to the middle of a plate and surround with the cucumber 'spoons', which children use to scoop up and eat the mash.

posh pockets

IF YOUR CHILD DOESN'T EAT WHEAT, USE ICEBERG LETTUCE LEAVES INSTEAD OF THE PITTA BREAD AND GIVE HIM OR HER OATCAKES OR OTHER WHEAT-FREE CRACKERS TO EAT ALONGSIDE.

½ ripe ***avocado****, peeled*
4 mini wholemeal pitta breads
½ ***cucumber****, thinly sliced*
8 small slices of smoked ***salmon***

Mash the avocado flesh with a fork, then spread over the insides of the pitta breads. Pack each pitta with cucumber discs and a couple of slices of smoked salmon.

These little pockets make a great packed lunch and they can have all sorts of other things stuffed into them, such as tomatoes.

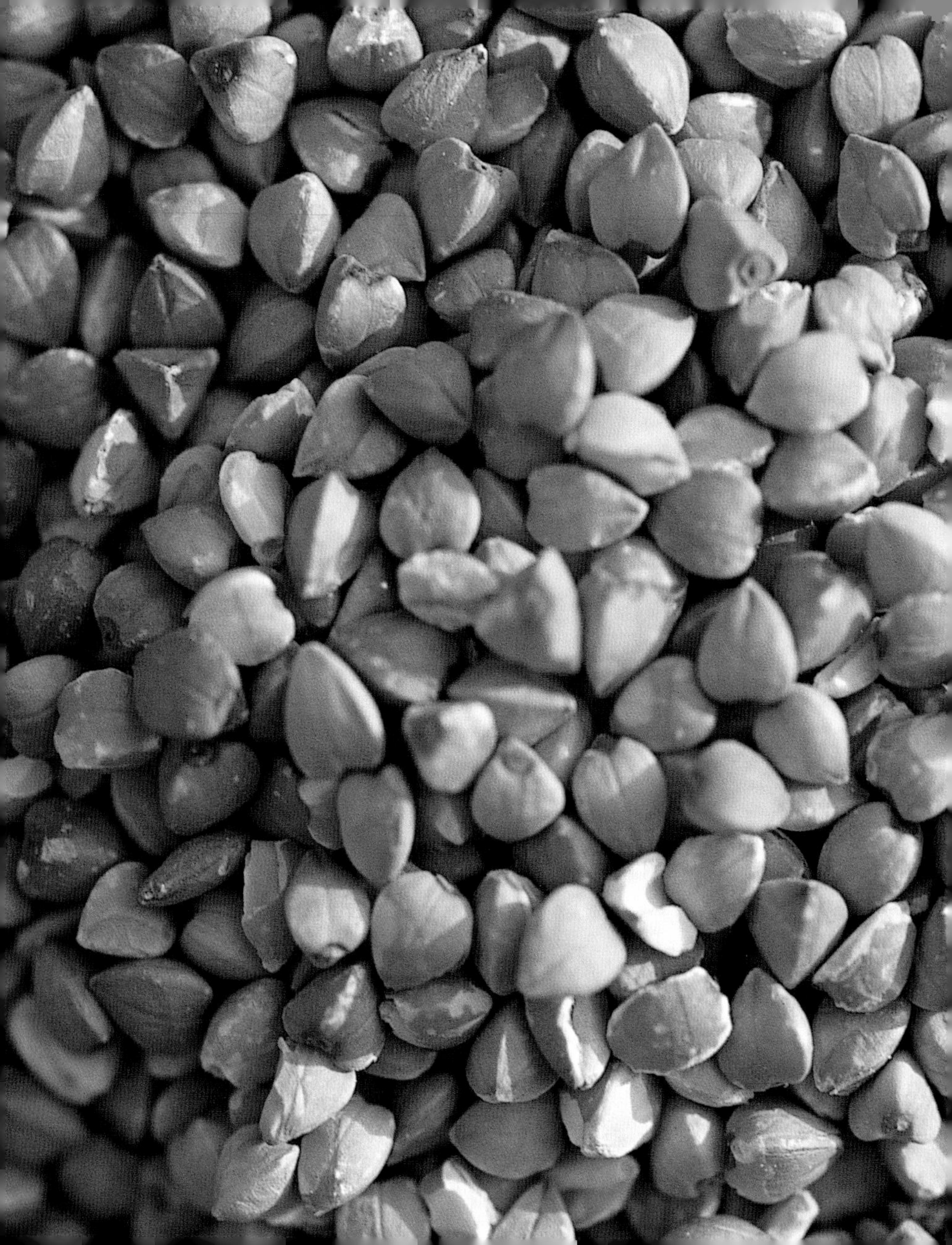

buckwheat

Despite its name, buckwheat is not related to common wheat, to which some children are severely allergic (as in coeliac disease) and some react on a milder level, with bloating or lethargy for example. Buckwheat doesn't contain gluten, the common offending substance in wheat but also in other grains such as oats, rye and barley. Studies comparing buckwheat to refined wheat have shown it is able to satisfy hunger better and also produce a much more desirable blood sugar and insulin response – all great for energising children without increasing their risk of becoming overweight or diabetic. Buckwheat is a source of the powerful antioxidant, rutin, which helps extend the all-important activity of vitamin C. It contains good levels of the mineral magnesium, which is considered the 'relaxing' mineral in terms of the nervous system and muscle contraction, and is needed for healthy bones and good blood sugar balance. Buckwheat has a rich, nutty taste. It can be used in savoury dishes as an alternative to rice, or as porridge, while the flour is used to make soba noodles, pancakes and in baked goods.

noodle soup

FOR CHILDREN WITH A WHEAT SENSITIVITY, USE 100% SOBA NOODLES HERE, I.E. ONES MADE ENTIRELY WITH BUCKWHEAT. YOU CAN USE READY COOKED CHICKEN, TURKEY OR INDEED ANY MEAT OR FISH, PRAWNS OR TOFU IF YOU PREFER.

3 boneless ***chicken*** *breasts, skinned*
1 tsp olive oil
1 tbsp sweet chilli sauce
2 ***garlic*** *cloves, peeled and crushed*
1.5 litres water
2.5cm piece fresh root ***ginger****, peeled and grated*
2 lemongrass stalks, sliced
1 ***carrot****, peeled*
2 spring ***onions****, trimmed*
2½ tbsp ***miso*** *paste*
*100g dried soba (****buckwheat****) noodles*
handful of mangetout
juice of ½ ***lime***
4 dashes of ***sesame*** *oil*

Cut the chicken into 1cm thick strips. Heat the olive oil in a large saucepan, add the chicken with the chilli sauce and garlic and toss over a medium heat until it is cooked through. (Cut open a piece to be sure.) Tip out on to a plate and keep it aside.

Then pour the water into the pan, add the ginger and lemongrass and bring to the boil. Lower the heat and simmer for at least 10 minutes. In the meantime, very finely slice the carrot and spring onions.

Using a slotted spoon, fish out the lemongrass bits from the pan (as most children won't like coming across them). Scoop out a mugful of the water, stir the miso paste into it, then pour back into the pan. Add the noodles, mangetout, carrot, spring onions and lime juice. Cook for about 6–8 minutes until the noodles are just tender.

Ladle the soup into serving bowls. Divide the chicken among them and drizzle a dash of sesame oil on top. This is one to eat straight away, not keep for later.

buckwheat salad

THIS IS AN ADAPTATION OF A SUMMER RICE SALAD MY MALTESE GRANDMOTHER USED TO MAKE FOR US TO TAKE TO THE BEACH FOR LUNCH, WHEN WE WERE SPENDING THE DAY THERE.

200g ***buckwheat***
200g can ***tuna*** *in brine, drained and flaked*
1 ***green pepper****, cored, deseeded and finely chopped*
4 spring ***onions****, trimmed and finely sliced*
3 hard-boiled ***eggs****, quartered*
12 olives, pitted and chopped
1 heaped tbsp capers
3 tbsp olive oil
juice of 1/2 ***lemon***
8 ***mint*** *leaves, finely chopped*
freshly ground black pepper
pinch of sea salt
3 large ***tomatoes****, roughly chopped*

Cook the buckwheat in boiling water (as you would rice) until tender. Tip into a sieve and refresh under running cold water; drain well.

Tip the cooled buckwheat into a large bowl, add all the other ingredients except the tomatoes and toss together. (Small children can help here.)

Only add the tomatoes just before eating, and if you don't think you're going to eat all the salad in one go, add them to individual plates to keep the salad fresh-tasting.

NOTE Just leave out or replace anything your children don't like, perhaps capers or olives. Personally, I don't fancy eggs with this lot but they're part of Nanna's original recipe!

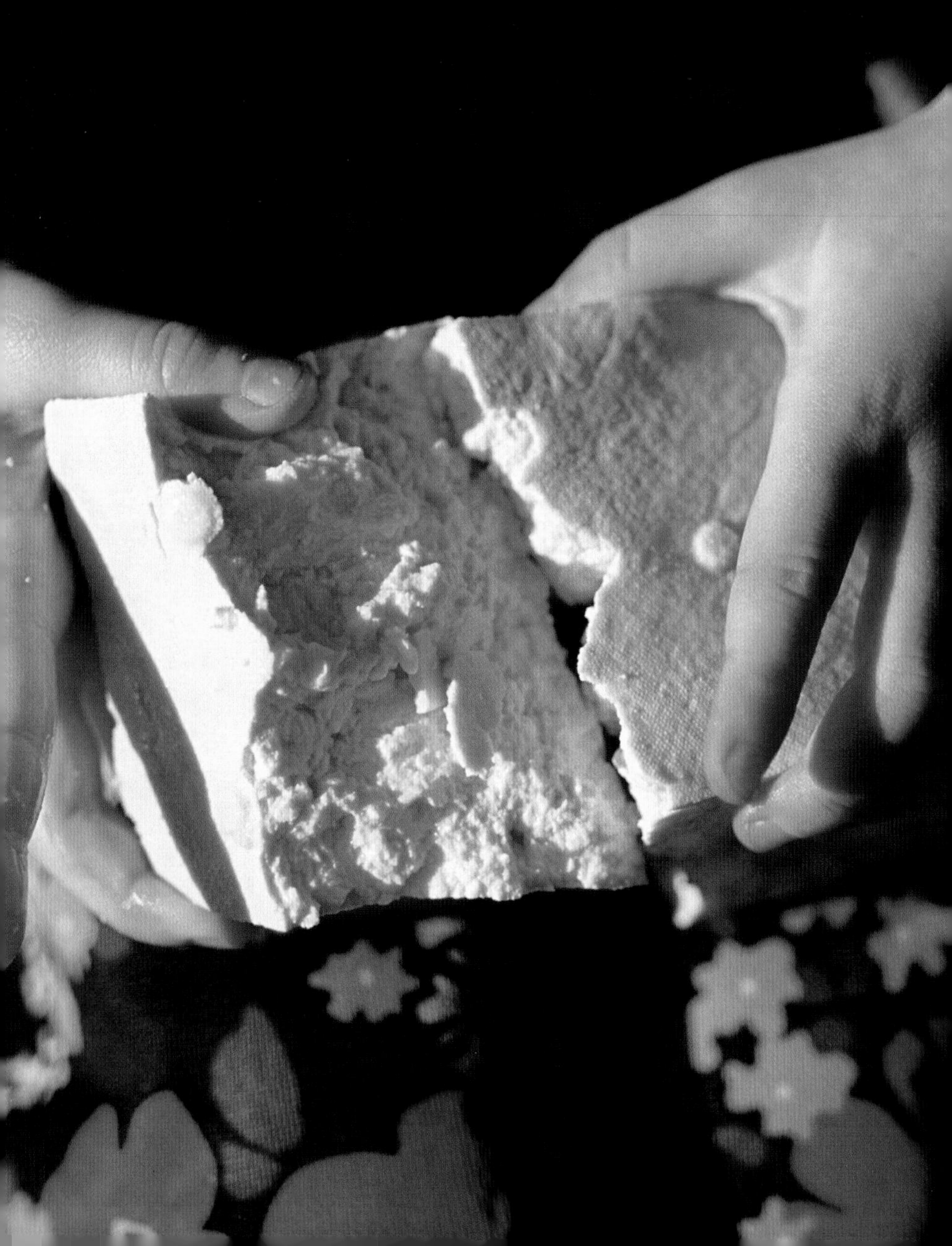

soya

Soya (and its derivatives) has been hailed both as a saviour and a demon. In one camp, it's a godsend for those intolerant of dairy produce, a vegetarian staple and a defender of hormones. In the other, it's notorious in highly processed foods derived from genetically modified beans that harm hormone balance. The truth probably lies somewhere between. Soya is, indeed, a viable alternative in the form of milk and yoghurt to dairy foods – ideal for children who cannot tolerate cows' or other animals' milk. It has also been shown to help lower cholesterol and enhance bone health. For vegan and vegetarian children, soya is a valid choice of protein (excluding the dodgy faux meat products that are highly processed). Because of its potential to affect hormone balance, it should be given to children in moderate amounts, say three or four servings a week; at this level it's probably beneficial. If your child cannot tolerate dairy foods, alternate soya with other 'milks' such as rice or almond. And buy organic to avoid genetically modified soya, or that grown on what was once pristine South American rainforest.

mighty berry slurpie

THIS MAKES A WONDERFUL BREAKFAST IN ITSELF, OR AT LEAST A SUBSTANTIAL MID-MORNING OR AFTERNOON SNACK. ON A HOT SUMMER'S DAY, ADD ICE CUBES FOR A WELL-CHILLED, REFRESHING 'SLURPIE'.

handful of ***blueberries***
handful of ***blackcurrants***
handful of ***strawberries****, hulled*
1 ripe ***banana***
6 tbsp plain ***soya yoghurt***
200ml ***apple*** *juice*
handful of ice cubes (optional)

Whiz all the ingredients together in a free-standing blender until smooth. (Young children can help by plopping the fruit into the blender).

Pour the 'slurpie' into tall tumblers and serve.

NOTE You can use frozen or canned berries (in juice, not syrup) if that's easier.

sesame stir-fry

A VARIATION ON THE THEME OF A BASIC STIR-FRY, DELICIOUS SERVED ON TOP OF RICE OR SOBA NOODLES.

200g firm ***tofu***
1cm piece fresh root ***ginger****, peeled and grated*
1 ***garlic*** *clove, peeled and grated*
1 tbsp sweet chilli sauce
1 spring ***onion****, trimmed*
handful of ***green beans***
1 ***carrot****, peeled*
½ ***red pepper****, deseeded*
1 tbsp olive oil
1 tsp Chinese five spice powder (optional)
1 tbsp tamari (or soy sauce)
2 tbsp water
2 tbsp ***sesame seeds***

Slice the tofu into strips and toss in a bowl with the ginger, garlic and chilli sauce; set aside.

Roughly slice the spring onion and green beans. Cut the carrot into thin strips and the red pepper into slightly thicker ones.

Heat a wok or frying pan, add the olive oil, with the Chinese five spice powder if using, and stir for a minute, then add the prepared vegetables. Toss quickly over a high heat for 4–5 minutes, adding the tamari and water to 'steam-fry' the veg.

Tip the veggie stir-fry into a warm bowl, then add the tofu mixture to the wok and toss quickly for a couple of minutes until it is heated through and nicely sticky on the outside.

Serve the stir-fried vegetables and tofu on noodles or rice, sprinkled with the sesame seeds.

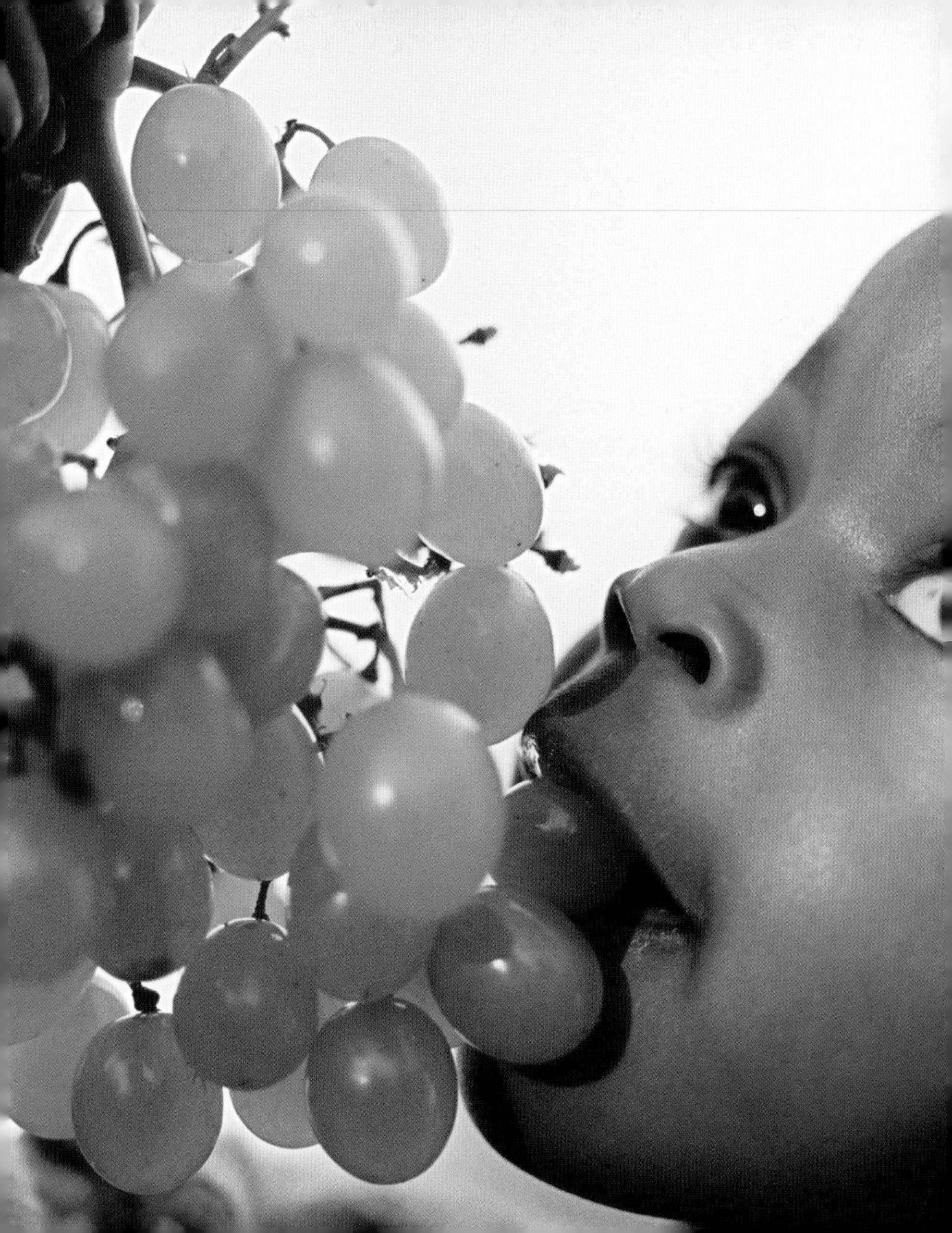

grapes

As children, my cousins and I were spoiled by our Auntie Anne (a patient nun!) who would painstakingly peel and deseed a cup of grapes for each of us. A rare treat, but actually, not one that did us the most favours in terms of the fibre and vitamins lost in the grape skins. The little, fingerfood aspect of grapes makes them a perennial favourite with children and they are certainly a healthy between-meal snack and dessert. Red grapes in particular, are loaded with powerful antioxidants such as quercetin and pterostilbene, which boost immunity, helping keep allergies calmed and more serious illnesses at bay. Much of the research into the health properties of grapes has focused on heart-protective and anti-cancer substances, which may seem less relevant for children but nevertheless are still important. Grapes, as you can tell from the shrinkage when they become raisins, are loaded with water. This and their fibre make them useful for cleansing the gut and preventing constipation. The sugar in grapes is easily absorbed, which makes them good for triggering a burst of energy.

goaty grape salad

NOT A GOAT IN SIGHT HERE FOR THIS TASTY, CHEESY SALAD, WHICH MAKES A LOVELY LUNCH SERVED WITH A SLICE OF RYE TOAST.

200g firm goat's cheese (any you like)
2 Little Gem lettuces, roughly torn
12 seedless red ***grapes****, halved*
12 seedless white ***grapes****, halved*
1 tbsp olive oil
1 tbsp cider vinegar
2 tbsp ***apple*** *juice*
freshly ground black pepper
2 tbsp ***pumpkin seeds***

Cut the goat's cheese into cubes or crumble it into pieces. In a large bowl, toss the lettuce, grapes and goat's cheese together.

Mix the olive oil with the cider vinegar and apple juice in a cup to make a dressing. Drizzle over the salad and toss to mix.

Sprinkle the salad with the pumpkin seeds just before you serve it up.

grape gobstoppers on a stick

THESE MAKE FUN, FROZEN 'LOLLIES'. THE LARGER THE GRAPES THE BETTER AND YOU COULD ADD OTHER TYPES OF FRUIT TOO.

12 seedless red ***grapes****, halved*
12 seedless white ***grapes****, halved*

Get the children to 'thread' six grapes on to each of four wooden kebab sticks, alternating the colours. Lay them on a tray lined with greaseproof paper and put them into the freezer for at least 4 hours.

Give them to the children as ice lollies that they can nibble and suck for some time.

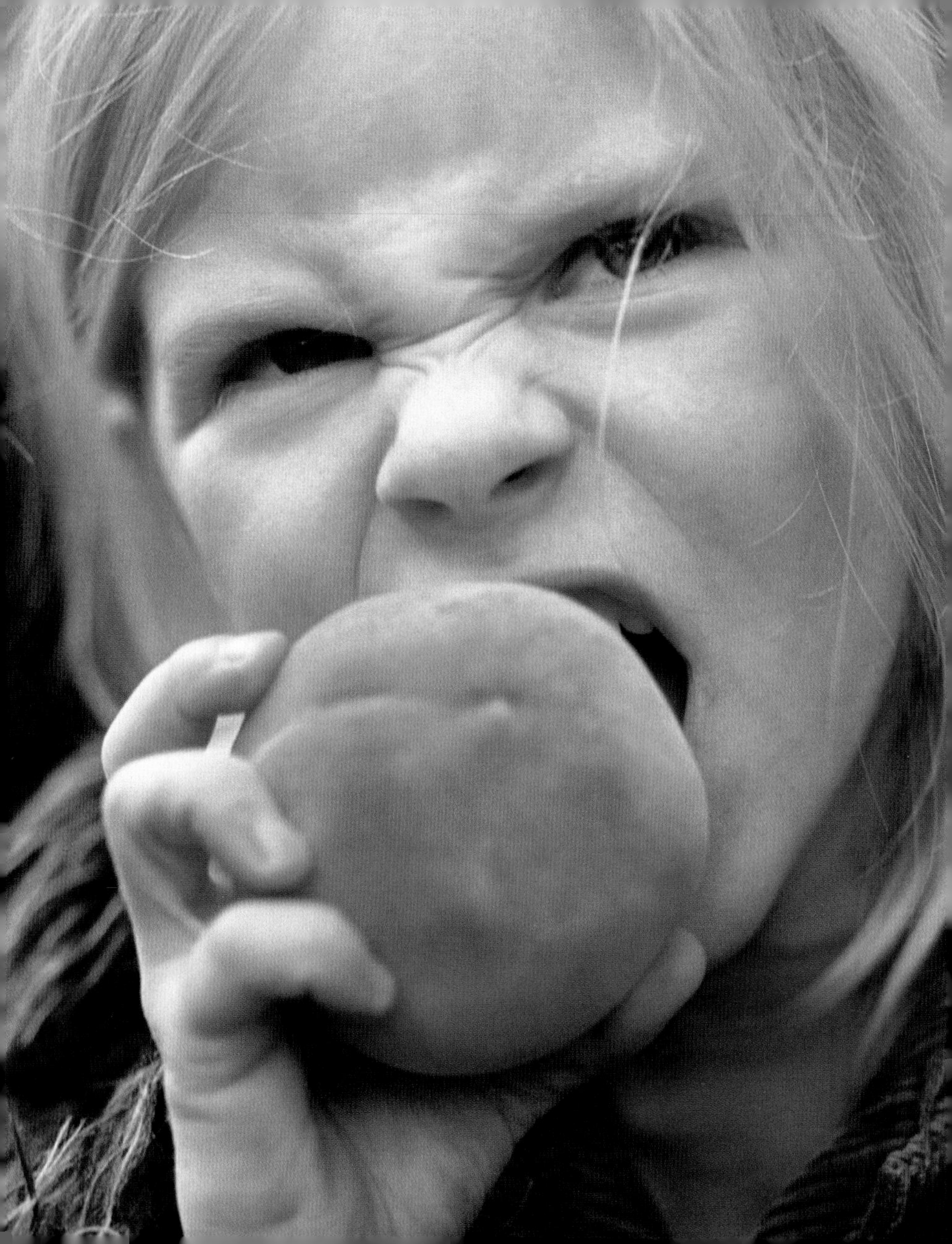

nectarine & peach

The names alone conjure up deliciousness – nectar, peachy, pretty as a peach... The syrupy sweetness of a ripe, fuzzy peach or smooth nectarine is one of summer's true delights. The flavour coupled with the goodness in these fruits makes them perfect treats that most children will enjoy. When ripe, they are easily digestible and tend to have a low allergy potential. Opt for nectarines if the fuzz on peaches puts your children off, as removing the skin diminishes the nutrient value. Their rich fibre and water content make both fruit good gut cleansers, relieving constipation and clearing wastes, especially important in children who have gut symptoms to food intolerances. Yellow-orange fleshed peaches and nectarines have a higher source of antioxidants than white-fleshed ones, particularly carotenes which are important for smooth, clear skin as well as a strong immune system and healthy lungs. Dried peaches make a sweet, healthy snack for children that is even more densely loaded with fibre and beta carotene than the fresh variety, although eating too many will create bloating and wind.

coconut rice pud with nectarines

IN THAILAND DURING APRIL, ROADSIDE STALLS SELL COCONUT RICE WITH FRESH MANGOES. THIS IS A VARIATION THAT I THINK COMES CLOSE TO MATCHING THE REAL THING.

150g ***brown rice***
1 tbsp ***sesame seeds***
200ml ***coconut*** *milk*
2 tbsp ***honey*** *or sugar*
3 ripe ***nectarines****, halved, stoned and sliced*

Cook the brown rice as directed on the packet. Meanwhile, in a dry frying pan over a medium heat, shake the sesame seeds until they are lightly toasted – carefully so as not to let them burn. Tip them on to a plate and leave them aside to cool.

When the rice is cooked, drain if necessary, then add the coconut milk and honey to the pan and stir over the heat for about 10 minutes. You end up with a mass of gooey rice.

Let the rice cool a little before serving in small bowls, topped with slices of fresh nectarine and sprinkled with the toasted sesame seeds.

peach slice

I TOP THIS POLENTA BASE WITH DIFFERENT FRUITS EACH TIME. IT'S GREAT SERVED WITH YOGHURT OR SOURED CREAM.

100ml ***apple*** *juice*
400ml water
2 tbsp ***honey*** *or maple syrup*
4 ***peaches****, sliced*
150g polenta or cornmeal
1 tsp butter
a little olive oil
about 20 ***almonds****, roughly broken up*

Preheat the oven to 180°C/Gas 4. Put the apple juice, water and honey into a large saucepan and bring to the boil. Turn down the heat and add the peach slices. Leave to simmer for 4–5 minutes, then remove the peaches with a slotted spoon and set aside on a plate.

Slowly add the polenta to the liquor in the pan over a medium heat, whisking constantly to avoid it getting lumpy. Whisk in the butter. Continue to cook the polenta until it is very thick and easily comes away from the sides of the pan – about 10 minutes, stirring regularly.

Rub the bottom of a 23cm flan dish with olive oil, pour in the polenta and bake in the oven for 30 minutes. Lay the peach slices on the polenta and scatter the almonds over the top. Put it back in the oven for 15 minutes.

Serve warm or cold, cut into slices.

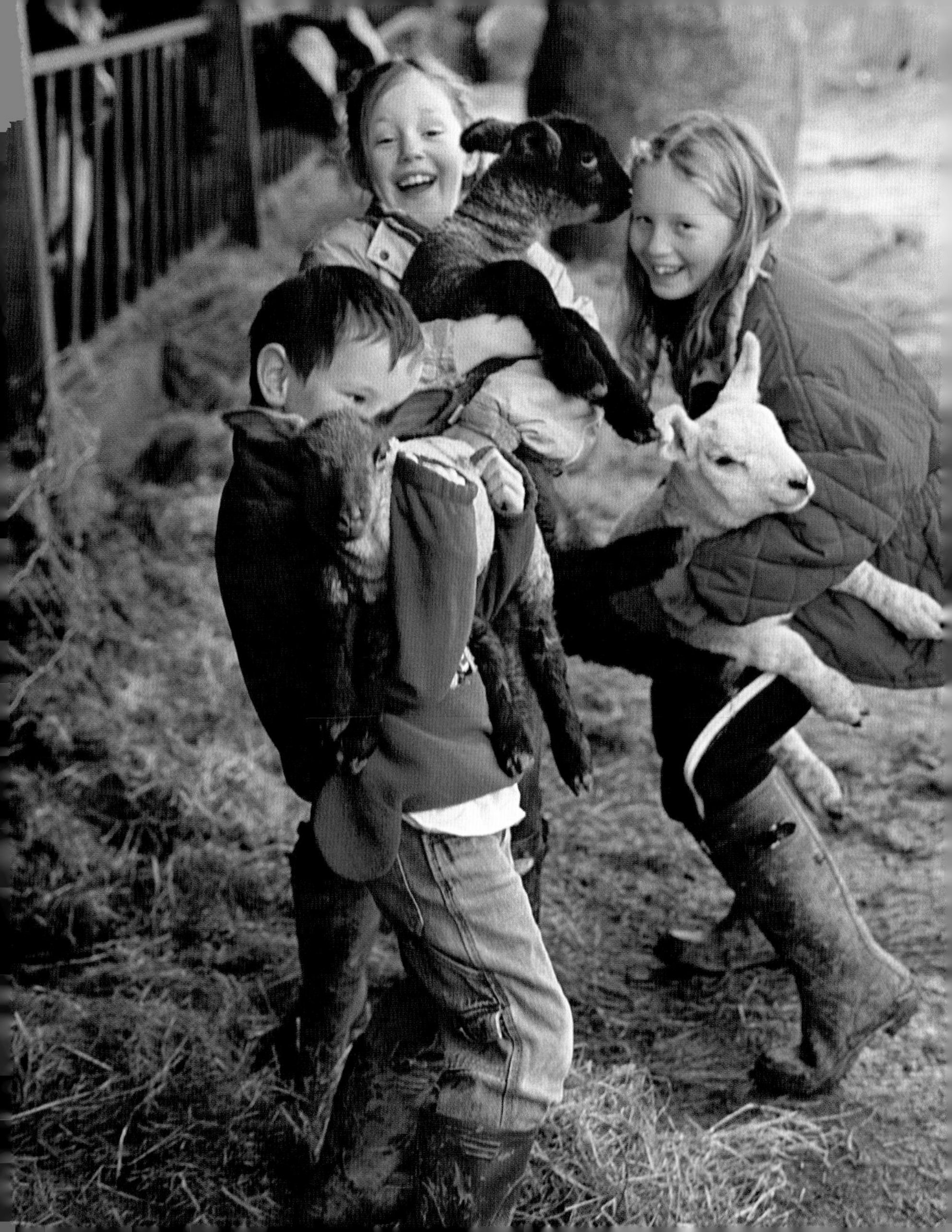

lamb

Many children don't even make the link between meat on their plates and cute, woolly lambs '*baaing*' in a field – if they've even seen them. Perhaps not a bad thing if you want your children to eat the meat! Lean, quality lamb, or indeed other lean meat, is a valuable part of an omnivore's diet. By definition, lamb comes from a younger animal that most likely grazed outdoors, in contrast with other intensively reared meat. From the allergy point of view, lamb tends to be one of the most tolerable, dense sources of protein for people who are highly reactive. Lamb, like all meats, is a good source of the mineral zinc, which is needed for proper growth in children and strong defences, as well as for cuts to heal. It also contains B vitamins, especially B_{12} which is only found in significant amounts in animal-derived foods and is needed for healthy growth, energy production and maintaining good moods. Meats such as lamb are rich in iron, important for carrying oxygen around the body to make energy and for girls at the onset of their menstrual cycles.

lamb burgers

THESE TAKE NO TIME AT ALL TO PREPARE AND ARE ABSOLUTELY DELICIOUS. YOU COULD MAKE DOUBLE AND FREEZE HALF TO COOK FOR ANOTHER MEAL.

500g lean ***lamb****, minced*
½ medium ***onion****, peeled and grated*
squeeze of ***lemon*** *juice*
1 tbsp ***rosemary*** *leaves, finely chopped*
1 tsp ground cumin
1 tsp ground ***cinnamon***
1 tbsp tamari (or soy sauce)

Put all the ingredients in a large bowl and mix together using your hands until evenly combined. Using wet hands, form the mixture into burgers, patting them into shape. (Young children can help here.) This amount should make about eight.

Preheat the grill or barbecue, then cook the burgers for about 4–5 minutes each side.

Serve them with Veggie rosti (page 162) or tucked into a wholemeal pitta bread with sliced tomatoes, cucumber and lots of salads.

NOTE Another delicious way of serving these burgers is sandwiched between two quickly fried, giant flat mushrooms.

kebab rolls

THE ONLY 'KEBAB' THING ABOUT THESE IS THE MEAT, OTHERWISE THEY'RE MORE LIKE CHINESE DUCK PANCAKES AND ALL THE MORE FUN FOR ROLLING YOUR OWN. CHINESE/VIETNAMESE RICE PANCAKES ARE AVAILABLE FROM MOST LARGE SUPERMARKETS AND ASIAN GROCERS, BUT IF YOU CAN'T FIND THEM USE MINI TORTILLAS OR CABBAGE LEAVES (AS FOR LEAF ROLLS, PAGE 85) INSTEAD.

300g ***lamb*** *fillet*
½ medium ***onion****, peeled and grated*
2 ***garlic*** *cloves, peeled and crushed*
1 tsp ground cumin
1 tsp Chinese five spice powder (optional)

FOR THE YOGHURT SAUCE
4 tbsp natural ***yoghurt***
juice of ½ ***lemon***
1 tbsp chopped ***mint*** *leaves*
pinch of sea salt

TO SERVE
3 medium ***tomatoes****, sliced*
about 12 rice pancakes

Slice the lamb into 1cm thick strips and toss with the onion, garlic, cumin and Chinese five spice powder if using, in a large bowl. Cover and leave to marinate in the fridge for at least 20 minutes, longer if you can.

Meanwhile for the sauce, mix the yoghurt, lemon juice, chopped mint and salt together. Lay out the tomato slices on a serving plate. Prepare the rice pancakes as directed on the pack.

Heat a griddle or frying pan until it is very hot, then add the lamb with its marinade. Cook, turning the meat regularly, for about 4 minutes. Transfer to a warm serving plate.

Get the children to make the kebab rolls: spread the pancakes with some minty yoghurt sauce, add a little lamb and some tomato slices and roll up. Eat straight away.

juicy chops

THESE ARE BASICALLY ROASTED LAMB CHOPS THAT STAY DELICIOUSLY MOIST AND MAKE THEIR OWN 'SAUCE' AS THEY COOK.

8 small ***lamb*** *chops*
1 courgette, trimmed
1 ***red pepper****, halved, cored and deseeded*
16 cherry ***tomatoes***
2 ***garlic*** *cloves, peeled and crushed*
1 tbsp ***honey***
1 tbsp Worcestershire sauce
1 mugful of boiling water
pinch of sea salt
freshly ground black pepper
handful of ***mint*** *leaves*

Preheat the oven to 190°C/Gas 5. Lay the lamb chops in a roasting pan. Cut the courgette into 2cm thick slices and the red pepper into 2–3cm squares. Scatter these around and over the chops, adding the tomatoes and garlic.

Stir the honey and Worcestershire sauce into the mugful of boiling water, add the salt and some pepper, then pour it over the lamb. Tuck in the mint leaves. Cook in the oven for 20–25 minutes until the chops are tender. Serve with Spotty mash (page 81).

easy roast lamb

A ROAST NEEDN'T BE A BIG PALAVER – THIS ONE IS EFFORTLESS. IT'S ALWAYS BEST TO COOK AN EXTRA BIG LEG SO YOU HAVE LEFTOVERS FOR PACKED LUNCHES OR SUPPER THE NEXT DAY.

1 leg of ***lamb****, about 2kg*
2 ***rosemary*** *sprigs*
1 ***onion****, peeled and sliced*
2 ***carrots****, peeled and sliced*
1 ***garlic*** *bulb, separated into cloves*
4 tbsp tamari
2 tsp coarse grain or Dijon mustard
1½–2 mugfuls of boiling water
freshly ground black pepper

Preheat the oven to 190°C/Gas 5. Trim any excess fat from the lamb. Lay the rosemary sprigs, onion and carrot slices in a roasting dish (ideally one with a lid) and sit the lamb on top. Scatter the garlic cloves (still in their skins) around the meat.

Mix the tamari and mustard together in a mug, top up with boiling water and pour over the lamb. Season with pepper, then put the lid on (if you have one).

Roast in the oven, allowing about 45 minutes per kg. Halfway through cooking, stir ½–1 mugful of boiling water into the juices in the roasting dish to make a tasty gravy. Leave the meat to rest in a warm place for about 15 minutes.

Slice the lamb off the bone and serve with the gravy, garlic and flavouring vegetables. Accompany with steamed broccoli or Sweet roast veg (page 45). Children can squish the soft garlic out of its skins straight into their mouths!

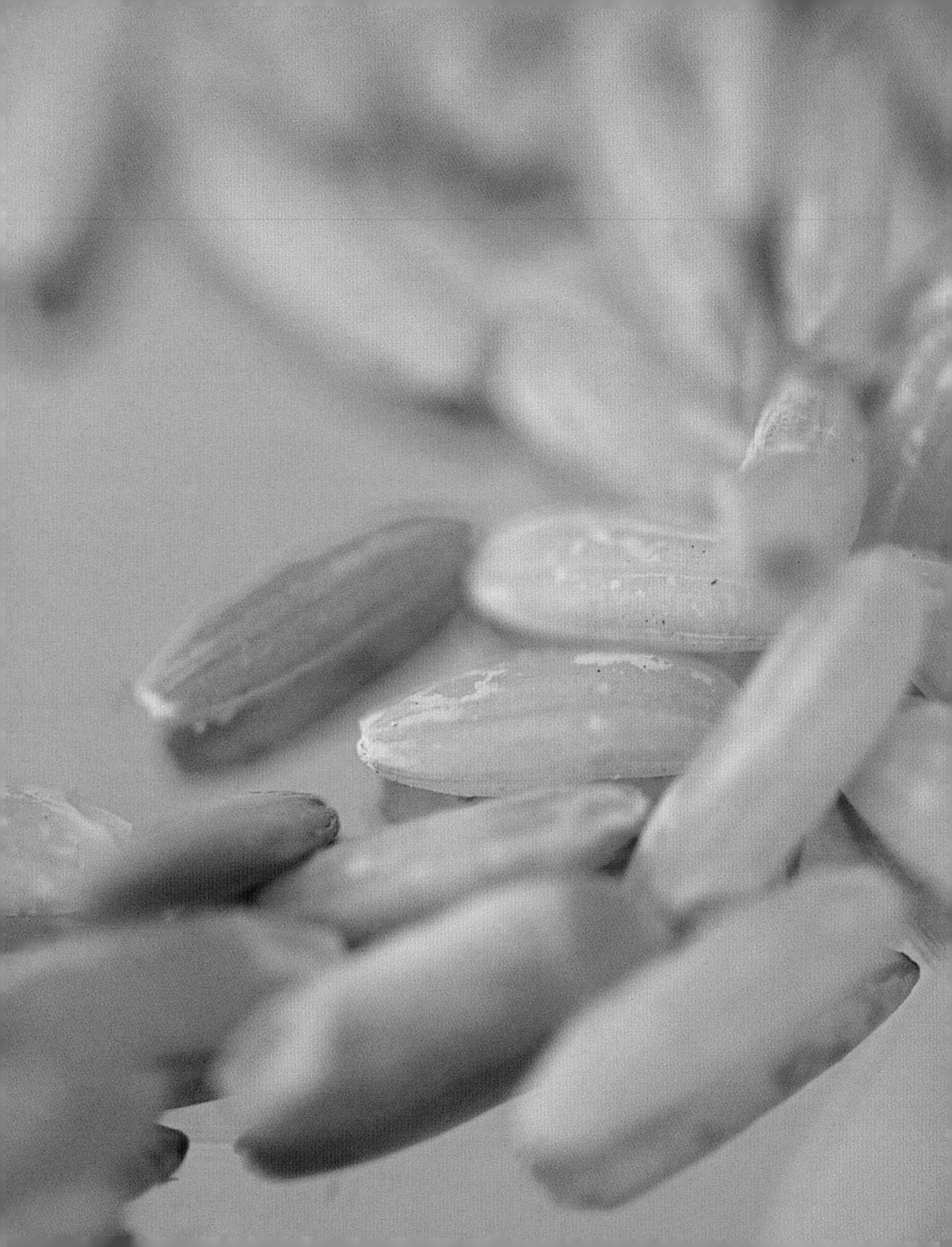

rice

At a time when more and more children are sensitive or allergic to wheat and other gluten-containing grains, rice is a popular, natural, inexpensive alternative. It is, after all, the staple grain for more than half of the people in the world and in the west it is commonly a baby's first grain food. Brown rice can be used as a base for sweet and savoury dishes, even though a generation back in this country, anything other than rice pudding was unthinkable. While a child with a very sensitive digestion may find brown rice slightly harsher than white, it is packed with fibre and much more nutritious. Indeed, brown rice contains as much as six times more of nutrients such as magnesium, zinc, vitamin E and folic acid than white rice. Its fibre gently bulks out the stool, making it easier to pass and feeds the important beneficial bacteria in the intestines. It also makes sure a meal leaves your child feeling more satisfied for longer. A common mistake when first using brown rice is to undercook it, so follow packet instructions, even slightly over-cooking it if necessary to make it more digestible for children.

rice salad

I MADE THIS COMBO USING SOME COOKED BROWN RICE THAT WAS IN THE FRIDGE WHEN I NEEDED TO RUSTLE UP A QUICK LUNCH WHILE WRITING! SOME CHILDREN SAY THEY FIND BROWN RICE TOO CHEWY, BUT YOU CAN OVERCOME THIS IF YOU COOK IT FOR LONG ENOUGH. UNLIKE WHITE RICE, IT IS HARD TO OVERCOOK.

150g ***brown rice****, cooked*
2 spring ***onions****, trimmed and finely sliced*
150g feta cheese, crumbled
12 cherry ***tomatoes****, quartered*
1 tbsp olive oil
juice of $\frac{1}{2}$ ***lemon***
1 tbsp chopped ***mint***

Cook the brown rice as directed on the packet, allowing at least 35 minutes to be sure it is tender. Tip into a sieve and refresh under running cold water, draining well.

Put the rice into a large bowl and add all the other ingredients. Toss it all together, then serve.

NOTE If you don't think the whole lot will be eaten at once, add the tomatoes to each plate rather than the full thing, as they'll spoil before the rest.

VARIATIONS Try adding olives, capers, chopped peppers, other vegetables, tofu instead of feta... the possibilities are endless.

spanish seafood rice

THIS IS MY CHEAT'S VERSION OF A PAELLA. YOU COULD ADD SQUID AND ANY OTHER FISH YOU LIKE.

175g **brown rice**
550ml *vegetable or chicken stock*
1 *tsp ground* **turmeric**
200g *smoked* **haddock** *fillet (undyed), skinned*
8 *large raw prawns, shelled and deveined*
8–12 *mussels (optional), cleaned*
1 *tbsp olive oil*
1 **onion**, *peeled and finely chopped*
1 *tsp ground cumin*
2 **garlic** *cloves, peeled and chopped*
1 **red pepper**, *cored, deseeded and sliced*
2 **tomatoes**, *peeled and roughly chopped*
100g **peas** *(frozen is fine)*
2 *tbsp chopped* **parsley**

Put the rice in a pan with 450ml of the stock and the turmeric and bring to the boil. Lower the heat, put the lid on and simmer for about 35 minutes until the rice is cooked.

Meanwhile, cut the smoked haddock into cubes, checking for any small bones. Set aside with the prawns and mussels if using.

In a wok or large frying pan, heat the olive oil and cook the onion with the cumin until it is soft. Add the garlic and red pepper and cook, stirring, for 3–4 minutes. Add the tomatoes and cook for another minute or two.

Add the peas to the wok with the remaining 100ml stock. Simmer gently for another couple of minutes, stirring occasionally. Add the fish and shellfish with the chopped parsley and simmer for 4–5 minutes until it is cooked; discard any unopened mussels.

Serve a pile of rice on each plate topped with the seafood and sauce.

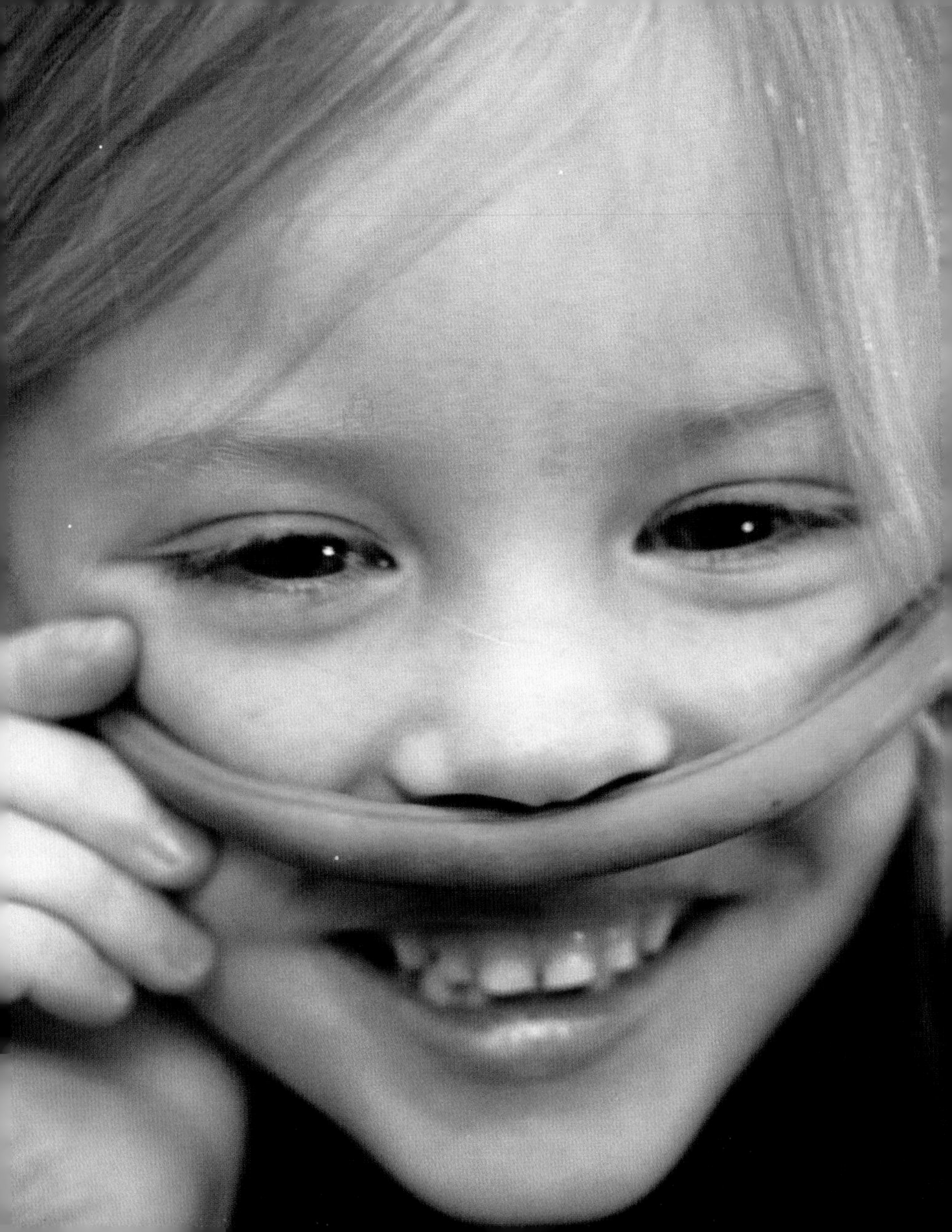

green beans

My appetite for green beans is a far cry from my childhood, when I insisted I hated them to the degree that my mother let me off their dreaded squeakiness. That was until the day she caught me happily scoffing them at my aunt's house. Now, their gentle flavour and soft but squeaky texture are all part of the attraction. It is rare for any green beans that you buy nowadays to have the unpleasant string that once gave them their name. Not only do green beans tend to be well tolerated, even by a sensitive gut, they are one of the best sources of the lesser-known vitamin K. This vitamin is essential for the body to make substances that help our blood to clot and also for children to build healthy bones during rapid growth stages. Green beans are also home to a host of other vital nutrients, including vitamin C, beta carotene, potassium, iron and fibre. If your children are averse to green beans, as I was, you will find they often go down well 'hidden' in a stir-fry or masked by other strong flavours, such as sesame.

green & white salad

THIS SIMPLE SALAD CAN BE EATEN WARM OR COLD AND MAKES A GREAT PACKED LUNCH. YOU CAN ADD OTHER INGREDIENTS, SUCH AS CELERY, TOMATOES, SPRING ONIONS... WHATEVER YOU FANCY.

2 boneless ***turkey*** *breasts, with skin*
1 tbsp olive oil
1 tbsp tamari (or soy sauce)
200g ***green beans****, topped and tailed*

FOR THE DRESSING
3 tbsp olive oil
1 tbsp cider vinegar
1 tsp Dijon mustard
pinch of sea salt

Preheat the oven to 190°C/Gas 5. Slice the turkey into 1cm thick strips, put into a small baking dish and add a little water, to just cover the bottom. Drizzle the olive oil and tamari over the turkey, cover with foil and bake for about 20 minutes until the turkey is cooked. Leave until cool enough to handle, then remove the skin.

Steam the beans or cook in boiling water for a few minutes until they are tender but not soft. Tip into a sieve and refresh under running cold water; drain well.

To make the dressing, shake the olive oil, cider vinegar, mustard and salt together in a jar.

In a large bowl, toss the turkey and green beans with the dressing, then serve.

sesame beans

A SIMPLE, DELICIOUS STIR-FRY, THAT DOESN'T DEMAND MUCH IN THE WAY OF CHOPPING. IF YOUR CHILD IS ALLERGIC TO SEEDS, USE OLIVE OIL, LEAVE OUT THE SESAME SEEDS AND ADD EXTRA GARLIC AND SOME CHOPPED HERBS SUCH AS CORIANDER OR PARSLEY FOR FLAVOUR.

2 tbsp ***sesame seeds***
1 tbsp ***sesame*** *oil*
2 ***garlic*** *cloves, peeled and crushed*
200g ***green beans****, trimmed and halved lengthways*
2 tsp tamari (or soy sauce)
2 tbsp water

In a dry frying pan or wok over a medium heat, toss the sesame seeds for a few minutes until they pop – take care that they don't burn, as this can happen very quickly. Tip them on to a plate and set aside to cool.

In the same pan, heat the sesame oil with the garlic for a minute. Throw in the beans and add the tamari with a splash of water. Stir-fry for about 5 minutes until the beans are cooked, but still a little crunchy.

Serve them sprinkled with the sesame seeds, as an accompaniment to a main dish, such as Dusted drumsticks (page 72).

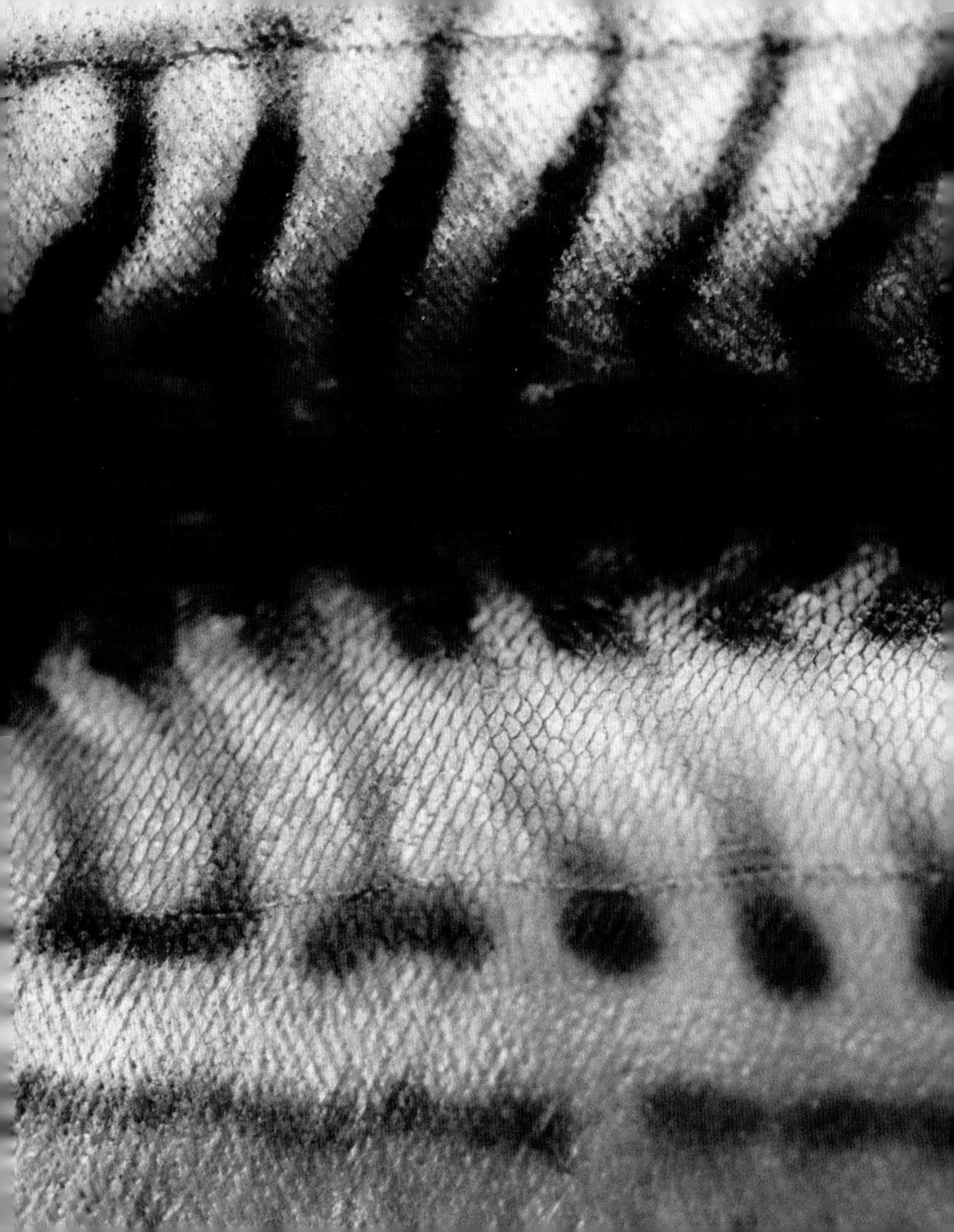

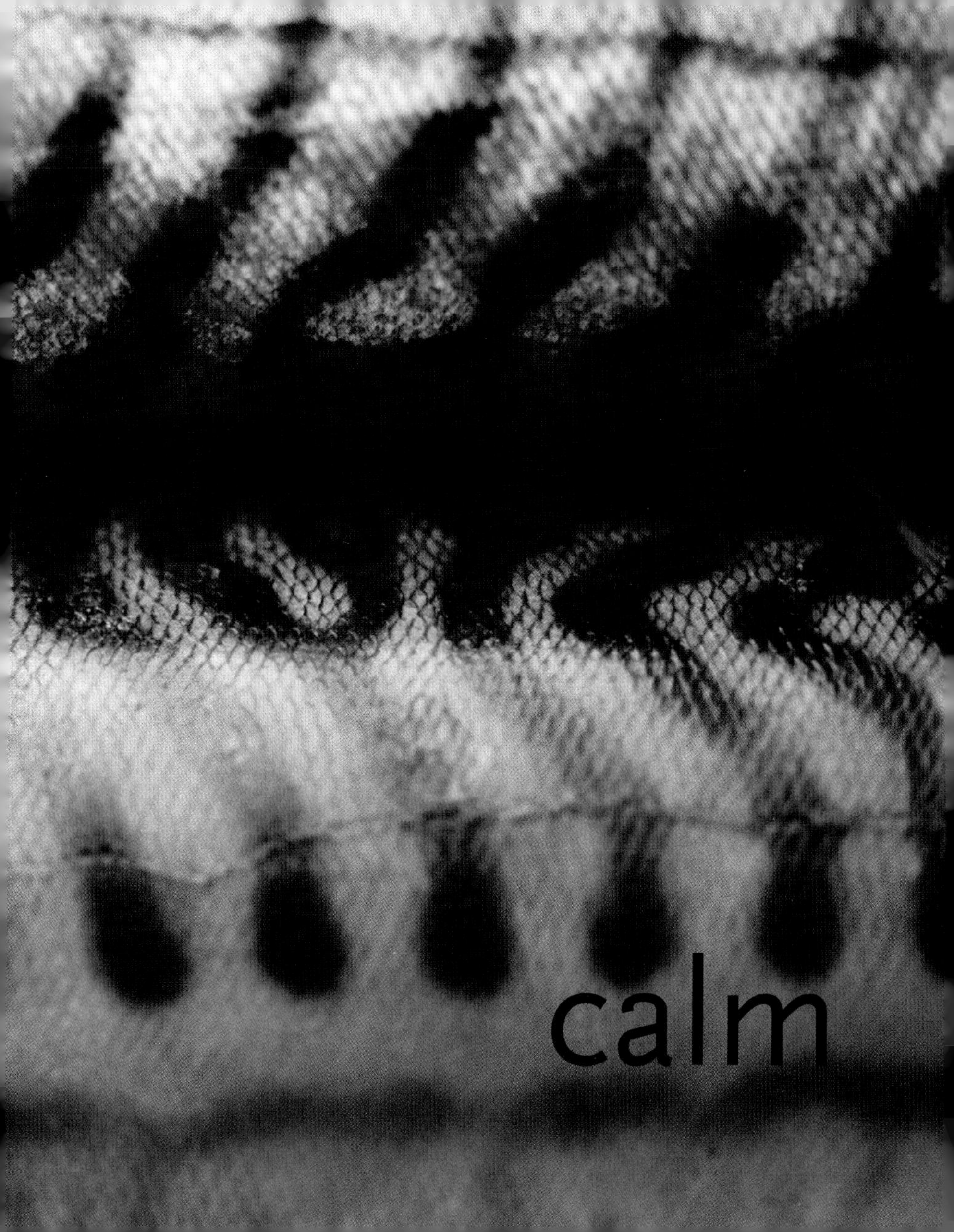

calm

Some of you may be disappointed to find out that the wonderfoods in this chapter are not going to subdue your little ones in order for you to get more peace and quiet. They are, however, foods that can help keep your children on an even keel both mood and energy-wise, and help them sleep well which ultimately makes life easier for you.

Some of the wonderfoods are here because they contain healthy fats, known to support a healthy nervous system. Oily fish, hemp seeds and linseed are all sources of important, polyunsaturated, essential fatty acids (EFAs). These fats not only help to make sure that the actual structure of nerve and brain cells are in good shape, they also enable the messages to bounce more efficiently from one nerve cell to the next. Scientific studies have shown that a good intake of these essential fatty acids is linked to a lower risk of depression and hyperactivity in children.

A key element in keeping mood and energy nicely balanced is blood sugar levels. If children are skipping meals or eating a lot of sugary or refined foods, their blood sugar levels are likely to seesaw, and with that, their vitality will fluctuate. To help maintain a more even blood sugar balance, you need to ensure your children eat regular meals that contain good quality protein, such as yoghurt, eggs or chicken, as well as other important elements like healthy, fibre-laden carbohydrates, such as quinoa or rye. Having protein, healthy fats and fibre at a meal ensures that the energy from food is not released rapidly, so your child has a gradual rather than sudden boost.

Several of the wonderfoods in this chapter contain an amino acid, a protein building block, called tryptophan. Turkey, chicken, yoghurt and seeds, for example, are good sources. In the body, as long as there are good supplies of other nutrients and enzymes, tryptophan can be converted into serotonin. This messenger molecule is linked to good moods and sleep. B vitamins and zinc are needed for serotonin production and these too are found in the wonderfoods in this chapter. Other nutrients associated with calming the nervous system are the minerals calcium and magnesium, both found in seeds, for example, and the former in yoghurt. Food sensitivities to additives as well as certain refined foods such as white flour can trigger mood changes in children – the foods here give you nutritious alternatives, for example, rye toast for breakfast instead of normal wheat bread.

A child's mood fluctuations or hyperactivity may be triggered or at least exacerbated by a number of factors not related to foods, such as unhappiness or feeling unsettled. It is therefore important to consider any issues that may be causing the disturbances, even ones that the child may not openly talk about. That said, if he or she is getting a broad-ranging, good intake of food, then at least your child has a great foundation on which to deal with other situations.

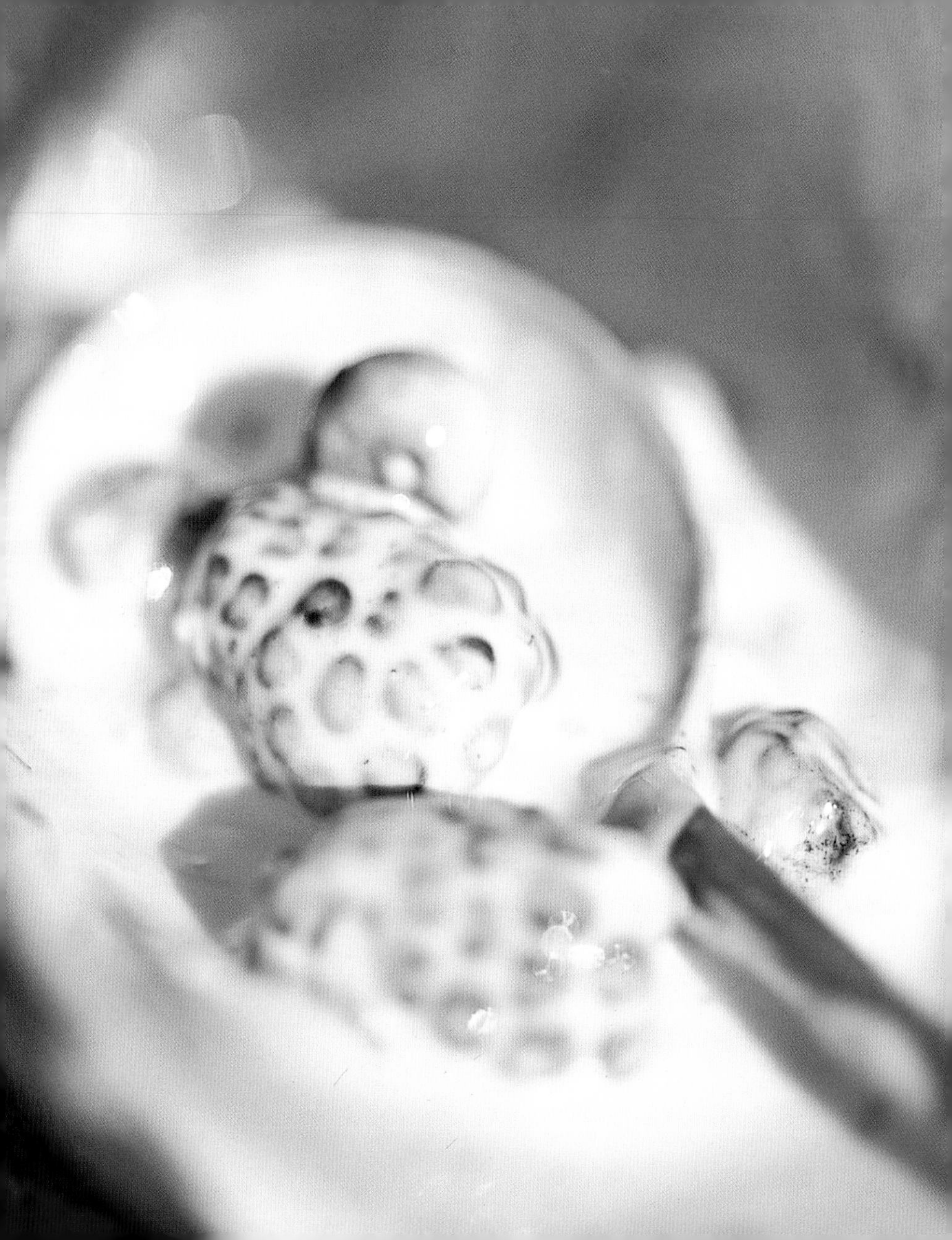

yoghurt

The yoghurt I'm referring to here doesn't include the cutely packaged, sweetened, colourful varieties marketed specifically to children. Most are laden with sugar and substances that change the texture – unnecessary in my view. Natural yoghurt has been a wonderfood for centuries, probably millennia, with ancient civilisations across the world valuing its qualities. Not only do your children benefit from the protein and calcium of milk in a more digestible form, but also the live bacterial cultures. These bacteria are responsible for keeping the immune system strong, aiding digestion, warding off tummy bugs, maintaining a healthy gut and replenishing the intestines after a course of antibiotics. Yoghurt contains a range of B vitamins needed for, amongst other things, balanced energy and temperament. The tryptophan in yoghurt is needed to produce the good mood neurotransmitter, serotonin. You can make natural yoghurt more appealing to children by adding fresh fruit or fruit purée, blending it in smoothies, stirring it into soups and sauces, or using it to top desserts.

pineapple lassi

THE ORIGINAL SMOOTHIE WAS PROBABLY A LASSI – AN INDIAN DRINK BASED ON NATURAL YOGHURT, SOMETIMES DRUNK AS A SAVOURY VERSION WITH SALT, GINGER AND SPICES. THIS FRUITY LASSI IS WONDERFULLY REFRESHING. SMALL CHILDREN CAN HELP TO MAKE IT BY MEASURING THE INGREDIENTS AND ADDING THEM TO THE BLENDER.

*½ **pineapple***
handful of ice cubes
*6 tbsp natural **yoghurt***
*100ml milk, **soya** milk or juice*
*3 tbsp **coconut** milk*
½ tsp ground mixed spice
*juice of ½ **lime***

Remove the peel and core from the pineapple, then cut into pieces. Put the pineapple and ice cubes in a free-standing blender and whiz until the ice is crushed and the pineapple is well pulped.

Add the other ingredients and blitz again for a minute, until well combined. Pour into four tumblers and serve.

mildly curried prawns

THE TASTY, GENTLE CURRY MARINADE USED HERE GOES WELL WITH ANY FISH, CHICKEN OR MEAT. YOU COULD EVEN PUT THE PRAWNS ON TO SKEWERS AFTER THEY'VE BEEN MARINATED TO COOK UNDER A GRILL OR ON A BARBECUE.

16 prawns, shelled and deveined
small handful of ***coriander*** *leaves*

FOR THE MARINADE
$\frac{1}{2}$ ***onion,*** *peeled and grated*
3 ***garlic*** *cloves, peeled and crushed*
1 tbsp olive oil
3 tbsp ***lemon*** *juice*
2 tsp ground cumin
1 tsp ground coriander
1 tsp paprika
2 tbsp grated ***coconut****, ideally fresh*
4 tbsp natural ***yoghurt***

Put all the ingredients for the marinade into a large bowl and mix well (young children could help here). Add the prawns and toss to coat them all over with the mixture. Leave the prawns to marinate for at least 20 minutes.

Tip the lot into a large frying pan and heat it up. Cook for 4–5 minutes until the prawns are pink and cooked through.

Serve the prawns in their sauce scattered with a few coriander leaves. Brown rice (perhaps boiled with a pinch of turmeric and a few cardamom pods) is the ideal accompaniment.

NOTE If you have the time and inclination, toast whole cumin and coriander seeds in a dry frying pan and grind them to a powder for the marinade.

VARIATION Cook some green veg, such as spinach leaves, in with the prawns and sauce too.

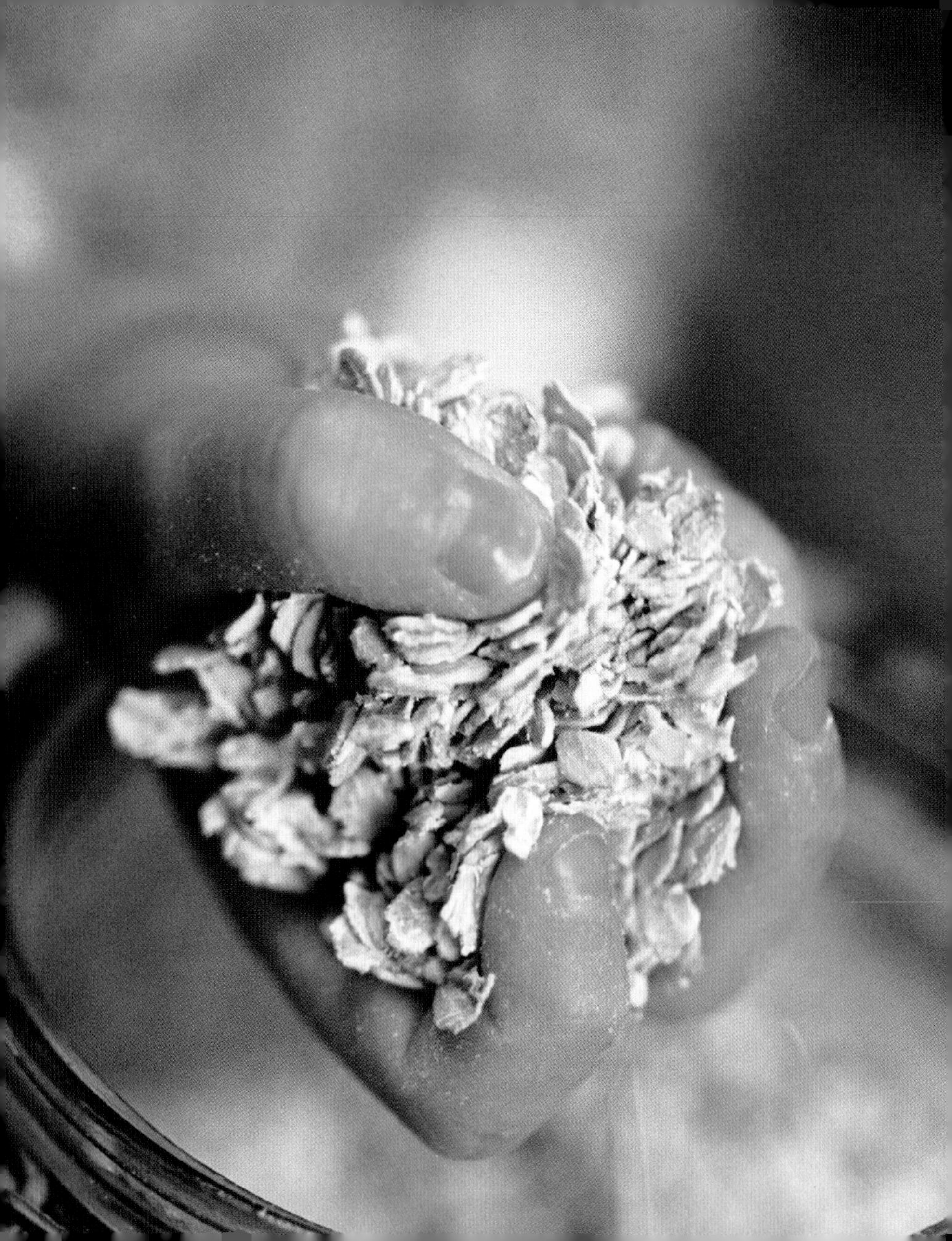

oats

Scientists have shown that children who eat breakfast are more likely to have better concentration, problem-solving skills and eye-hand co-ordination, and oats are ideal breakfast food. They are one of the best forms of carbohydrate you can feed your children because they come packaged with lots of fibre as well as vitamins and minerals. The fibre makes the release of energy from oats gentle rather than dramatic, so they help keep energy and mood level for a considerable time after they are eaten; hence their reputation as a long-lasting breakfast base. Oats contain a fibre-like substance called beta-glucan, which is gaining a reputation for boosting immunity and lowering cholesterol. An old folk remedy for reducing anxiety and depression is herbal tincture of oats. This wonderful grain is packed with energy-giving, mood-balancing B vitamins, vitamin E and vital minerals such as iron and zinc. Oats are more than just the ultimate breakfast food – they can be used to top sweet and savoury crumbles, to thicken soups and ground to make a 'biscuit' base for sweet and savoury tarts.

thick chicken soup

THE OATS MAKE THIS SOUP LOVELY AND THICK. IT IS REAL COMFORT FOOD – IDEAL FOR A COLD DAY. YOU COULD EVEN PUT SOME IN A FLASK FOR A PACKED LUNCH.

1 tbsp olive oil
2 ***onions****, peeled and sliced*
2.5cm piece fresh root ***ginger****, peeled and grated*
2 ***garlic*** *cloves, peeled and crushed*
2 celery sticks, finely chopped
1 ***carrot****, peeled and finely diced*
2 large, skinless ***chicken*** *breasts*
1.2 litres chicken stock
1 bay leaf
2 heaped tbsp medium ***oatmeal***
freshly ground black pepper
1 tbsp chopped ***parsley***

Heat the olive oil in a large saucepan and gently sweat the onions, ginger, garlic, celery and carrot for about 10 minutes.

Meanwhile, finely slice the chicken breasts. Add to the pan and cook for another 5 minutes or so, stirring occasionally.

Pour in the stock, add the bay leaf and bring to the boil. Stir in the oatmeal and a little pepper and lower the heat. Leave the soup to simmer for 10 minutes, then remove the bay leaf, stir in the parsley and serve.

NOTE If you do not have medium oatmeal, simply whiz porridge oats in a blender for a minute.

oaty veg crumble

THIS CRUMBLE IS A GREAT MAIN MEAL IN ITSELF, PERHAPS WITH SOME STEAMED BROCCOLI ALONGSIDE. YOU CAN CHUCK ANY VEGETABLES INTO IT – EVEN SOME COOKED CHICKEN OR PULSES IF YOU LIKE. FOR A FINER TOPPING, GRIND HALF OF THE OATS IN A BLENDER.

1 tbsp olive oil
3 ***garlic*** *cloves, peeled and crushed*
1 leek, trimmed and thickly sliced
2 ***carrots****, peeled and thickly sliced*
2 courgettes, thickly sliced
10–15 ***green beans****, cut into 1cm slices*
6–10 ***shiitake*** *or chestnut* ***mushrooms****, quartered*
400g can chopped ***tomatoes***
1 tbsp ***tomato*** *purée*
150ml water
1 tbsp chopped ***basil***
freshly ground black pepper

FOR THE TOPPING

250g porridge ***oats***
60g butter, diced
2 tbsp ***pumpkin seeds***
2 tbsp ***hazelnuts****, roughly crushed*
2 tbsp freshly grated Parmesan cheese

Preheat the oven to 190°C/Gas 5. Heat the olive oil in a large saucepan, add the garlic, leek and carrots and stir over a medium heat for 5 minutes. Add the courgettes, green beans and mushrooms and cook, stirring for a further 2–3 minutes.

Pour in the tomatoes, tomato purée and water, stirring well, then add the basil and season with pepper. Bring to the boil, cover the pan, lower the heat and simmer for 10 minutes.

To make the crumble, put the porridge oats in a bowl and rub the butter into them, using your fingertips. Mix in the pumpkin seeds, hazelnuts and Parmesan. (Even young children could be shown how to do this.)

Tip the vegetables into an ovenproof dish. Scatter the crumble mixture evenly over the top, patting it down so it reaches the edges of the dish. Bake in the oven for 35–40 minutes until the crumble topping is golden brown.

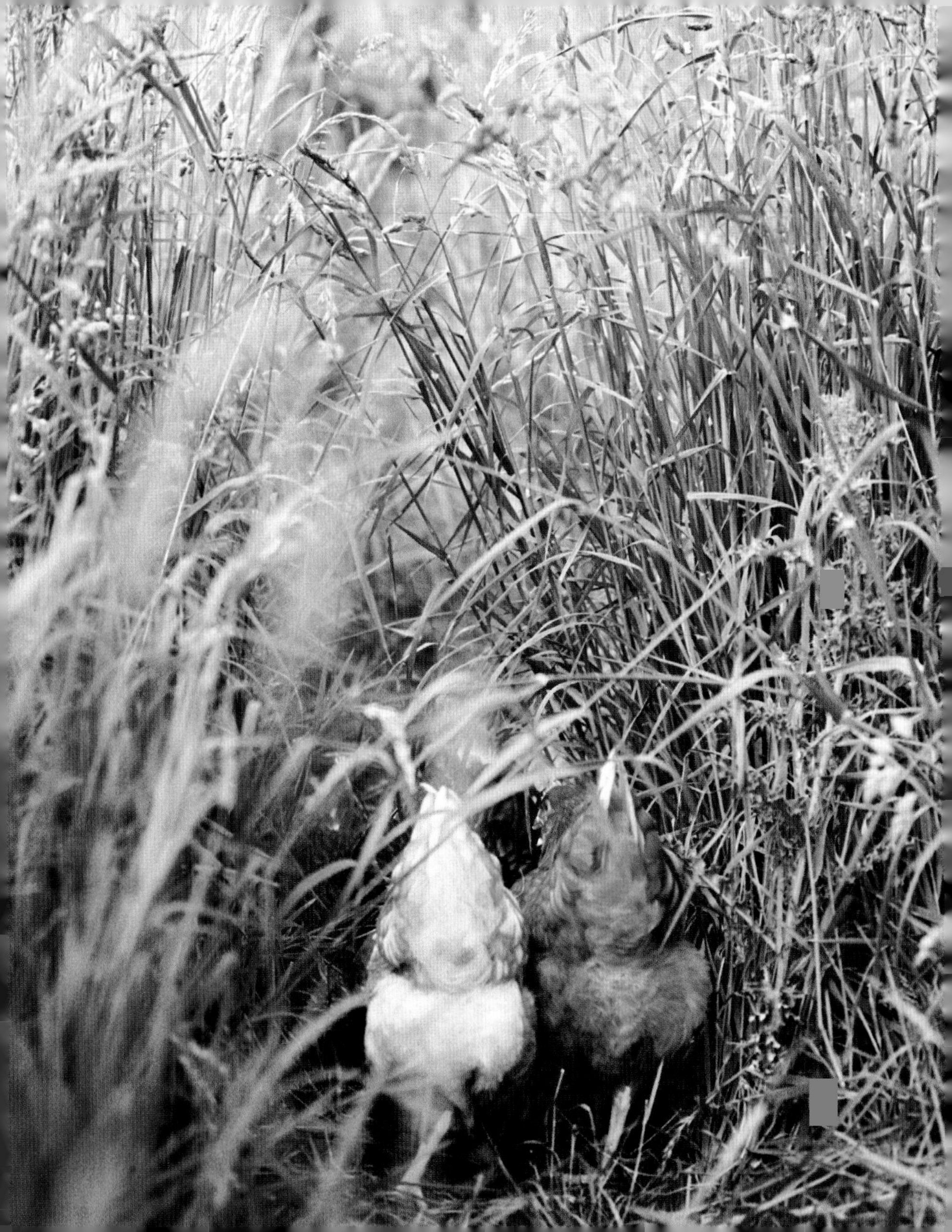

chicken & turkey

Most children love chicken and turkey, even if they don't know which way up the creature was when it was running around a yard, and even when it's not served alongside a mound of Christmas presents! Both meats are packed with nutrients for good balanced moods, including the amino acid, tryptophan, which can be converted in the body into the 'happy hormone' serotonin. In order for this to happen, it needs a good supply of vitamins B_3 and B_6, both of which are found in poultry. These vitamins are also needed for the body to make energy and help keep blood sugar levels balanced, a crucial factor in maintaining even moods and get-up-and-go (i.e. not slumping or becoming hyperactive). The mineral, zinc, in chicken and turkey is important for growth, immunity, skin health and healing as well as balanced moods. As a good source of low-fat protein, poultry provides good building blocks for growing, young bodies and makes a meal sustaining for children long after they've eaten it. Don't wait for Christmas to eat turkey, after all it was the first meal eaten on the moon in July 1969!

baked turkey rolls

THESE ARE SIMPLE AND DELICIOUS. YOU COULD USE THE HEMP PESTO (PAGE 156) HERE IF YOU HAVE SOME TO HAND.

2 large ***turkey*** *breasts, skinned*
2 tsp pesto sauce
4 slices Parma ham
1/4 ***pineapple***
1 tbsp tamari
1 mugful of water

Preheat the oven to 190°C/Gas 5. Lay the turkey breasts on a board and slice them in half horizontally. Lay the four slices flat on a board.

Children can help make the rolls: smear some pesto on each turkey slice and lay a slice of ham on top. Then roll up each one and secure it with a cocktail stick. Lay the rolls in a baking dish.

Remove the skin and core from the pineapple, then cut the flesh into cubes and scatter them around the turkey.

Stir the tamari into the mug of water and pour it around the turkey rolls. Cover the dish with a lid or foil and bake in the oven for 40 minutes. Serve the turkey rolls with Sweet roast veg (page 45) or Spotty mash (page 81).

sticky chicken

YOU CAN USE THIS 'STICKY SAUCE' TO MARINATE ANY MEAT OR FISH BEFORE GRILLING, BAKING OR COOKING ON A BARBECUE. IF YOU CAN'T GET HOLD OF SMOKED PAPRIKA, JUST LEAVE IT OUT. OLDER CHILDREN MAY LIKE A TOUCH OF CHILLI SAUCE ADDED.

*8 **chicken** drumsticks*

FOR THE MARINADE

*3 heaped tbsp **tomato** purée or ketchup*
1 tbsp balsamic vinegar
1 tbsp Worcestershire sauce
*2 tbsp runny **honey***
*2 **garlic** cloves, peeled and crushed*
1 tsp smoked paprika
2 tsp Chinese five spice powder (optional)

Mix the ingredients for the marinade together in a big bowl. Put the chicken pieces in, swishing them around so they are well coated. (A young child can help here, while an older one could manage the recipe alone.) Cover and leave to marinate for a couple of hours, or ideally overnight in the fridge.

Preheat the oven to 190°C/Gas 5. Put the drumsticks on a baking tray and roast them in the oven for 40 minutes until the chicken is cooked right through to the bone. Serve with Traffic light salad (page 277) or Spotty mash (page 81).

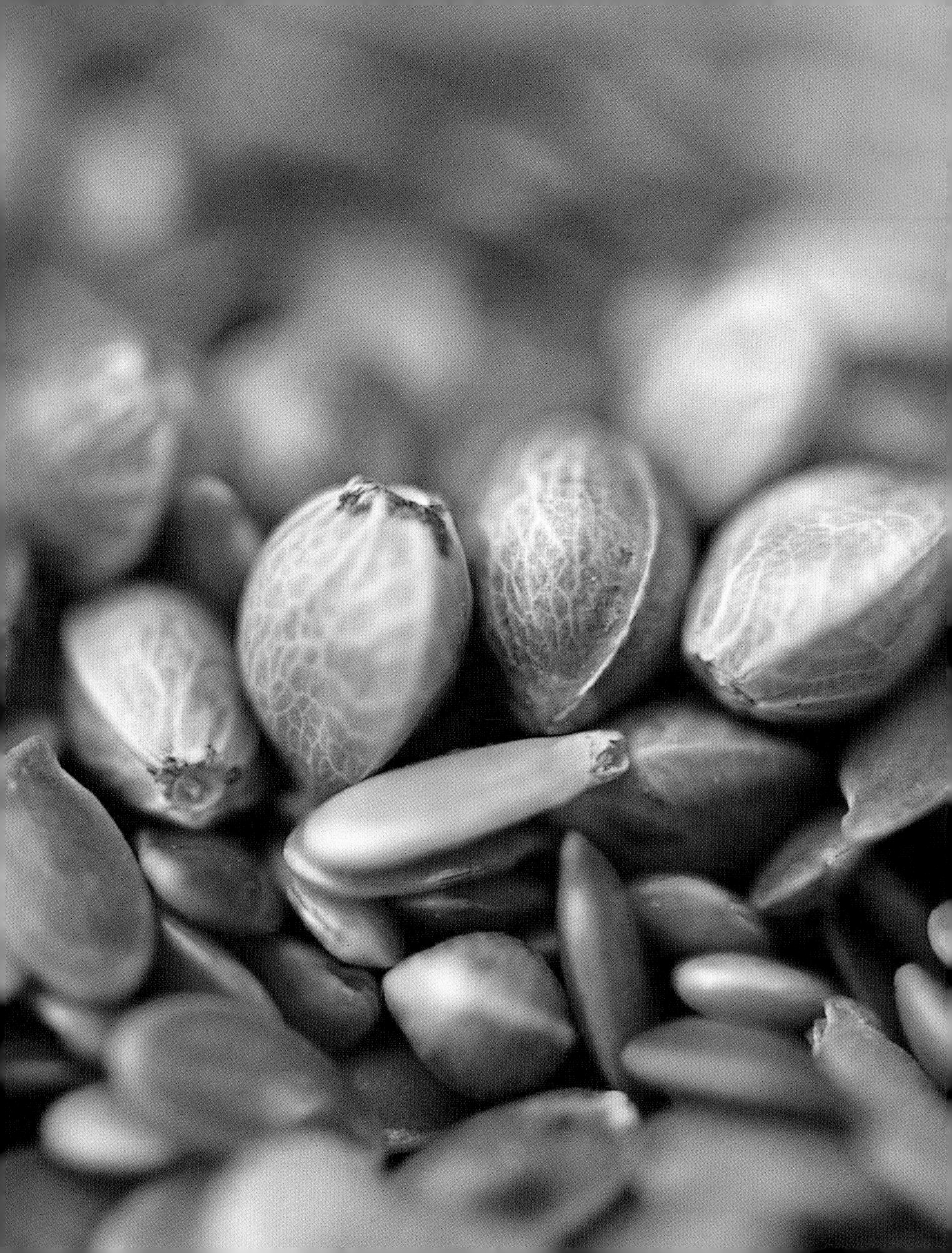

hemp seeds & linseed

Don't worry, you're not introducing your children to drugs (hemp is marijuana) or bird food (both seeds are given to budgies). Rather, to give them edible, human grade hemp and linseed is to expose them to near perfect wonderfoods. Both seeds are good sources of protein – especially important for vegetarian or vegan children. And the healthy fibre they contain not only feeds beneficial gut bacteria and helps prevent constipation but also clears waste products out of the body and makes a meal more sustaining in terms of energy release. As well as providing minerals like magnesium, hemp and linseed (and their oils) are wonderful sources of essential fatty acids. These EFAs have several vital roles in a child's body. They are needed for a healthy nervous system and brain, including the firing of messages for memory, learning and moods; smooth, supple skin; hormone messaging, such as girls' menstrual hormones and those that dictate metabolism; and alleviating conditions such as asthma and eczema. One EFA, called GLA has been linked to reducing hyperactivity symptoms in children.

hemp pesto

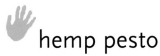

THIS DELICIOUS SAUCE NOT ONLY GOES WITH PASTA, LIKE A REGULAR PESTO, BUT ALSO WITH ANY GRILLED FISH OR MEAT.

6 tbsp ***hemp seeds***
2 ***garlic*** *cloves, peeled*
large handful of ***basil****,*
stems removed
150g Parmesan cheese,
finely grated
juice of 1/2 ***lemon***
freshly ground black pepper
3–4 tbsp olive oil (or more
if needed)

Whiz the hemp seeds, garlic, basil, Parmesan, lemon juice and pepper together in a free-standing blender, adding the olive oil a little at a time until you have a smooth, fresh sauce.

Toss the pesto with freshly cooked pasta or serve smeared over grilled fish or meat, or in Baked turkey rolls (page 152).

high five seed mix

THIS GROUND SEED MIX CAN BE EATEN AS A NUTTY TOPPING ON YOGHURT, CEREAL, SOUPS AND CASSEROLES. ALWAYS STORE SEEDS IN SEALED JARS IN A COOL, DARK PLACE AS THE ESSENTIAL FATTY ACIDS THEY CONTAIN ARE EASILY OXIDISED BY HEAT AND LIGHT.

equal quantities of:
hemp seeds
linseed *(flax seeds)*
pumpkin seeds
sunflower seeds
sesame seeds

Grind a batch of mixed seeds in a coffee grinder – ideally kept for the purpose! You can do a load in advance if you like, but keep the mix in an airtight jar in the fridge because once they're ground, the seeds are even more prone to rancidity.

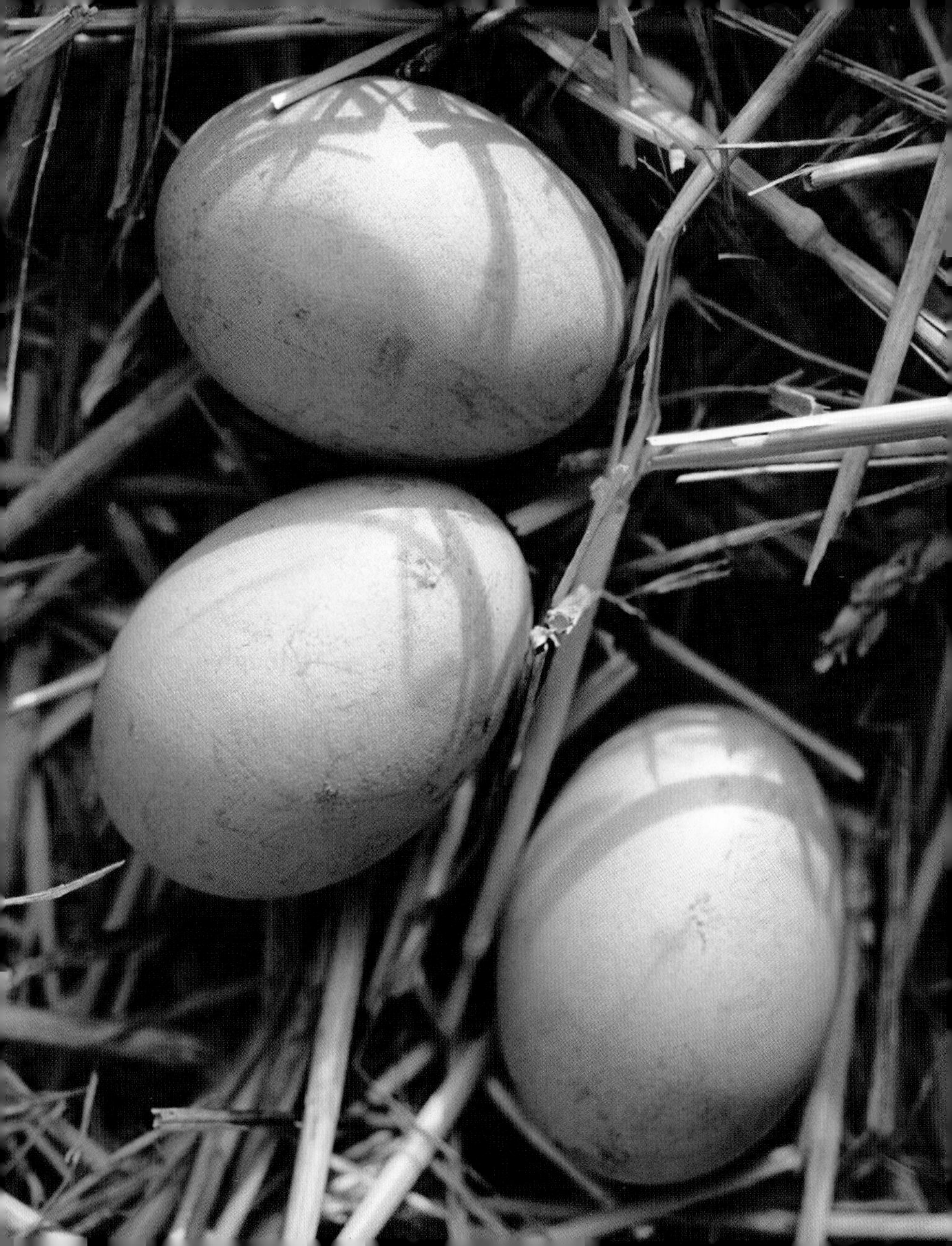

egg

A high quality, low-cost, protein-rich wonderfood in a shell, an egg goes way beyond its role as a dip for toasted soldiers. The dense protein in eggs provides the full range of essential building blocks for your child's growth and development. What's more, having such a protein in a meal means that the subsequent release of fuel is a measured one, leaving your child with a gradual supply of lasting energy. Although eggs get a rap for being high in cholesterol they contain more 'good' monounsaturated fat (as in olive oil) and anyway, cholesterol is needed for making stress and sex hormones and healthy cell membranes. Egg yolks also contain choline, which is used, amongst other things, to make acetylcholine, a crucial molecule in the brain responsible for memory and by extension, learning. For children, eggs are a good source of vitamin K, needed for proper blood clotting and bone formation, and selenium, the cancer-protective, antioxidant mineral. The goodness of an egg depends on the health and diet of the chicken that laid it, so always opt for organic, free-range eggs.

super scrambled eggs

THIS RICH, TASTY BREAKFAST TREAT GOES PERFECTLY ON HOT, LIGHTLY BUTTERED RYE TOAST WITH A GLASS OF ORANGE JUICE ON THE SIDE.

4 large ***eggs***
splash of milk or ***soya*** *milk*
freshly ground black pepper
knob of butter
125g smoked ***salmon*** *trimmings, finely diced*
1 large handful washed baby ***spinach****, chopped*
4 slices of hot toast, to serve

In a bowl, beat the eggs with a little milk and a grinding of pepper.

In a non-stick saucepan over a low heat, melt the butter. Swirl it around the bottom of the pan and add the eggs. Stir the eggs gently and as soon as they begin to set, add the smoked salmon and spinach. Keep stirring gently over a low heat for 3–4 minutes until the eggs are softly scrambled or the consistency you like, but certainly not until they turn rubbery.

Pile the scrambled eggs on to hot toast and serve straight away.

stop-go slice

YOU COULD MAKE THIS SPANISH OMELETTE FOR SUPPER AND REFRIGERATE ANY LEFTOVERS TO PACK INTO LUNCHBOXES THE NEXT DAY.

100g potatoes, scrubbed
6 ***eggs***
freshly ground black pepper
1 tbsp olive oil
1 courgette, thinly sliced
2 medium ***tomatoes,*** *skinned and sliced*
4–6 ***basil*** *leaves, torn*
2 tbsp freshly grated Parmesan cheese

Par-boil the potatoes in a pan of water for about 10 minutes, then drain and slice them into rounds when they are cool enough to handle.

Preheat the grill. Beat the eggs in a bowl with a little pepper. Heat the olive oil in a large non-stick frying pan over a medium heat and pour in the beaten eggs. Scatter the potatoes, courgette, tomatoes and basil over the egg and sprinkle with the Parmesan.

Cook, without stirring, for about 3 minutes on the hob, then put it under the hot grill for a minute or two until the omelette is golden brown on top. Serve cut into wedges.

NOTE Make sure your frying pan is suitable for placing under the grill.

veggie rosti

THESE FRITTERS ARE A GREAT WAY FOR CHILDREN TO ENJOY VEGETABLES. THEY GO WELL WITH ANY MAIN DISH, SUCH AS BAKED TURKEY ROLLS (PAGE 152).

1 large ***sweet potato****,*
peeled
1 large courgette
1 small ***onion****, peeled*
1 ***egg****, beaten*
pinch of sea salt
freshly ground black pepper
2 tbsp olive oil

Grate the sweet potato, courgette and onion, then drain on kitchen paper, squeezing out as much of the moisture as you can with your hands.

Tip the grated vegetables into a bowl, add the beaten egg, salt and some pepper and mix well. Shape the mixture into small patties using your hands (or small children could do this).

You'll need to cook the patties in batches. Heat the olive oil in a frying pan and lay the patties in the pan, flattening them slightly with a fish slice. Cook over a medium heat for about 5 minutes on each side. Remove and lay them on kitchen paper to drain while you cook the rest. Serve warm.

apple custard slice

THIS DESSERT IS VERY QUICK TO MAKE AND IS DELICIOUS HOT WITH SOURED CREAM, OR IT CAN BE EATEN COLD. YOU CAN USE EATING APPLES IN PLACE OF THE COOKERS, IN WHICH CASE IT WILL BE SWEETER.

2 large cooking ***apples****,*
peeled, cored and sliced
4 ***eggs***
300g natural ***yoghurt***
100g caster or brown sugar
2 tsp vanilla extract
1 tsp ground ***cinnamon***

Preheat the oven to 180°C/Gas 4. Lightly grease a 23cm flan dish. Peel, core and slice the apples.

Whisk all the other ingredients together in a large bowl until smooth.

Lay the apple slices evenly in the bottom of the flan dish, then carefully pour the whisked mixture over them (young children can do this).

Bake in the oven for 35–40 minutes until golden and firm. To test, insert a knife into the middle – it should come out clean. Cut into slices to serve.

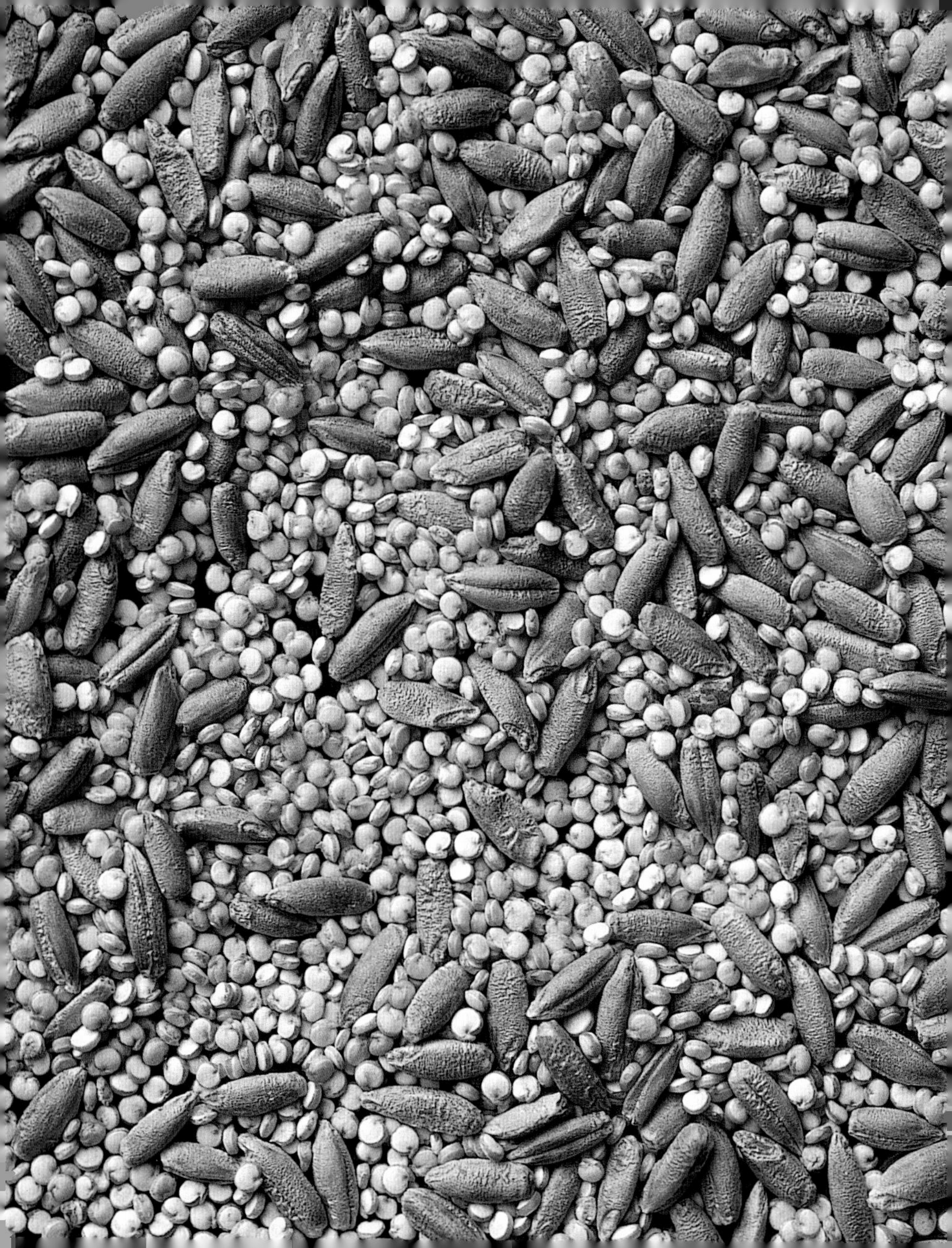

quinoa & rye

These intriguing grains may not have graced your kitchen, but both quinoa and rye are storehouses of nutrients. Quinoa's goodness is perhaps illustrated by the fact that it bears the name 'mother grain' in a native South American language. I love the way the grain separates when cooked to form what looks like a halo or a flying saucer! For a grain, quinoa is relatively rich in gluten-free protein, including the amino acid tryptophan, which can be made into the 'happy hormone' serotonin. It also provides a range of micronutrients, including B vitamins, iron, magnesium and manganese, packed in with the fibre and carbohydrate. Quinoa can replace couscous or rice in any dish. Rye is a hardy grain, usually sold in a relatively unrefined form leaving it high in fibre, which in turn leaves your child feeling more satisfied for longer and helps with gut health. Eating such foods makes children less likely to overeat and become overweight. Rye is most easily available in the form of rich, nutty rye bread, but the grains themselves and the flour can be put to good use in cereals and baking.

smart lunchbox sandwich

THERE'S NO REASON A QUICK SARNI OR LUNCHBOX STAPLE NEED BE UNHEALTHY OR BORING. EVEN YOUNG CHILDREN CAN MAKE THESE.

2 tbsp cottage cheese
100g cooked prawns, chopped
1 tbsp ***lemon*** *juice*
dash of Worcestershire sauce, to taste
8 slices of ***rye*** *bread*
4 large slices of smoked ***salmon***
2 medium ***tomatoes****, sliced*

In a bowl, mash the cottage cheese with the prawns, lemon juice and Worcestershire sauce. Spread this mixture evenly on the slices of bread.

Lay the smoked salmon and tomato on half of the bread slices and top with the others to make four smart sandwiches.

spiced quinoa & coconut fish

YOU COULD USE PIECES OF CHICKEN, LEAN MEAT OR PRAWNS INSTEAD OF THE FISH FOR THIS. DON'T BE PUT OFF BY THE LONG LIST OF INGREDIENTS, IT'S QUICKER THAN IT LOOKS TO PREPARE. YOU COULD, OF COURSE, JUST MAKE THE SPICED QUINOA TO EAT, HOT OR COLD, WITH ANOTHER MAIN COURSE.

1 mugful of ***quinoa****, rinsed*
½ tsp ground ***turmeric***
10 ***cardamom*** *pods*
1 ***cinnamon*** *stick*
2 tbsp ***raisins***
2 mugfuls of water
FOR THE COCONUT FISH
1 tbsp olive oil
1 ***onion****, peeled and finely sliced*
1cm piece fresh root ***ginger****, peeled and grated*
2 ***garlic*** *cloves, peeled and crushed*
12 ***almonds***
2 tsp ground ***cinnamon***
1 tsp ground coriander
300g chunky firm, white ***fish*** *fillet, such as monkfish, cubed*
juice of 1 ***lime***
200ml ***coconut*** *milk*
pinch of sea salt

Put the quinoa, turmeric, cardamom, cinnamon and raisins in a saucepan. Pour in the water, stir and bring to the boil, then lower the heat. Cover the pan and leave to simmer gently for 15 minutes.

Meanwhile, prepare the coconut fish. Heat the olive oil in a large frying pan and sauté the onion, ginger, garlic, almonds and spices for about 5 minutes. Add the fish with the lime juice and fry, turning the fish cubes until they are well coated with spices. Pour in the coconut milk, add the salt, stir gently and leave it to simmer for 15 minutes.

Discard the cinnamon and cardamom pods from the quinoa then pile on to plates. Top with the fish and coconut sauce and serve some steamed green veg on the side.

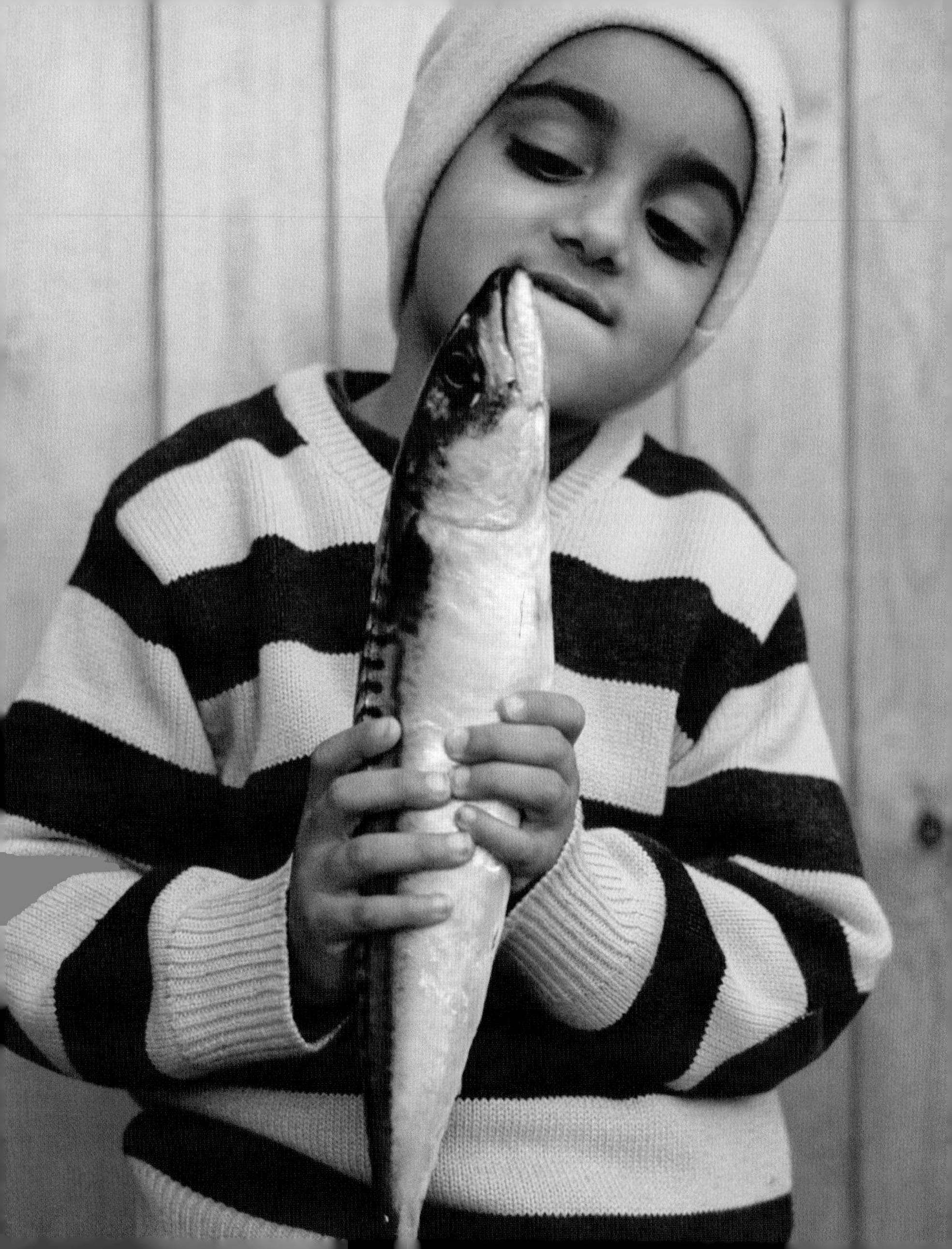

oily fish

It's not surprising that oily fish are renowned as brain food for children. Salmon, sardines, herring, mackerel, trout, fresh tuna – all are rich sources of the omega 3 essential fatty acids (EFAs), EPA (eicosapentaenoic acid) and DHA (docosahexaenoic acid). These confer a range of benefits, not least in healthy brain and nerve cell structure. If the membranes of such cells are in good shape, then neurotransmitters (messengers) for memory, learning and mood fire more efficiently. Because EPA and DHA are meshed into all cell membranes, they help keep skin soft and supple, which is particularly important in conditions such as eczema, where their anti-inflammatory properties are also called into play. Such properties are useful in other allergic conditions too, assuming that your child tolerates fish. Healthy cell membranes containing EFAs mean cells respond better to hormones such as insulin, helping maintain even blood sugar levels, helping balance energy and reducing the likelihood of obesity or diabetes. Fish also contains choline, the precursor to acetylcholine, needed for memory and learning.

smoked mackerel pâté

THIS IS A SUPER-QUICK, EASY PÂTÉ THAT CAN GO IN LUNCHBOX SANDWICHES. I SOMETIMES MAKE IT BY JUST MUSHING IT ALL UP WITH A FORK IN A BOWL.

150g smoked ***mackerel*** *fillet*
1 spring ***onion****, trimmed and roughly chopped*
110g cottage cheese
3 tbsp water
juice of ½ ***lemon***
1 tbsp chopped ***parsley***

Break the fish up, checking for any small bones as you do so. Put it into a free-standing blender and add the other ingredients. Whiz it all together until you have a pâté the consistency your children like – very smooth or with more texture.

Put the pâté into a bowl and chill in the fridge until you're ready to serve it up. It's lovely on crackers or warm bread, sprinkled with a squeeze of lemon juice.

salmon satay

THESE LITTLE SKEWERS MAKE A WONDERFUL MEAL IN THEMSELVES. YOU COULD ADD CUBES OF TOFU OR USE THEM INSTEAD OF THE SALMON, OR SUBSTITUTE CHICKEN OR LEAN MEAT FOR A CHANGE.

2 ***salmon*** *fillets, about 300g in total, cut into chunks*
4 raw prawns, shelled and deveined

FOR THE SATAY SAUCE
2 tbsp peanut butter
8 ***almonds***
1 ***tomato***
3 tbsp water (or more)
1 small ***garlic*** *clove, peeled*
1–2 tsp tamari (or soy sauce), to taste
2 tbsp ***lime*** *juice*
dash of Tabasco (optional)

To make the satay sauce, mix all of the ingredients together, using a hand-held stick blender until you have a smooth, thin sauce – add more water if necessary. Put it into a serving bowl.

Preheat the grill to high. Thread the fish chunks and one prawn on to each of four wooden skewers (small children could do this).

Place the fish under the grill and cook for 5–6 minutes, turning them a few times, until the fish is cooked through and the prawns are pink.

Serve the skewers with the peanut sauce, accompanied by Sesame beans (page 137) and brown rice or rice noodles.

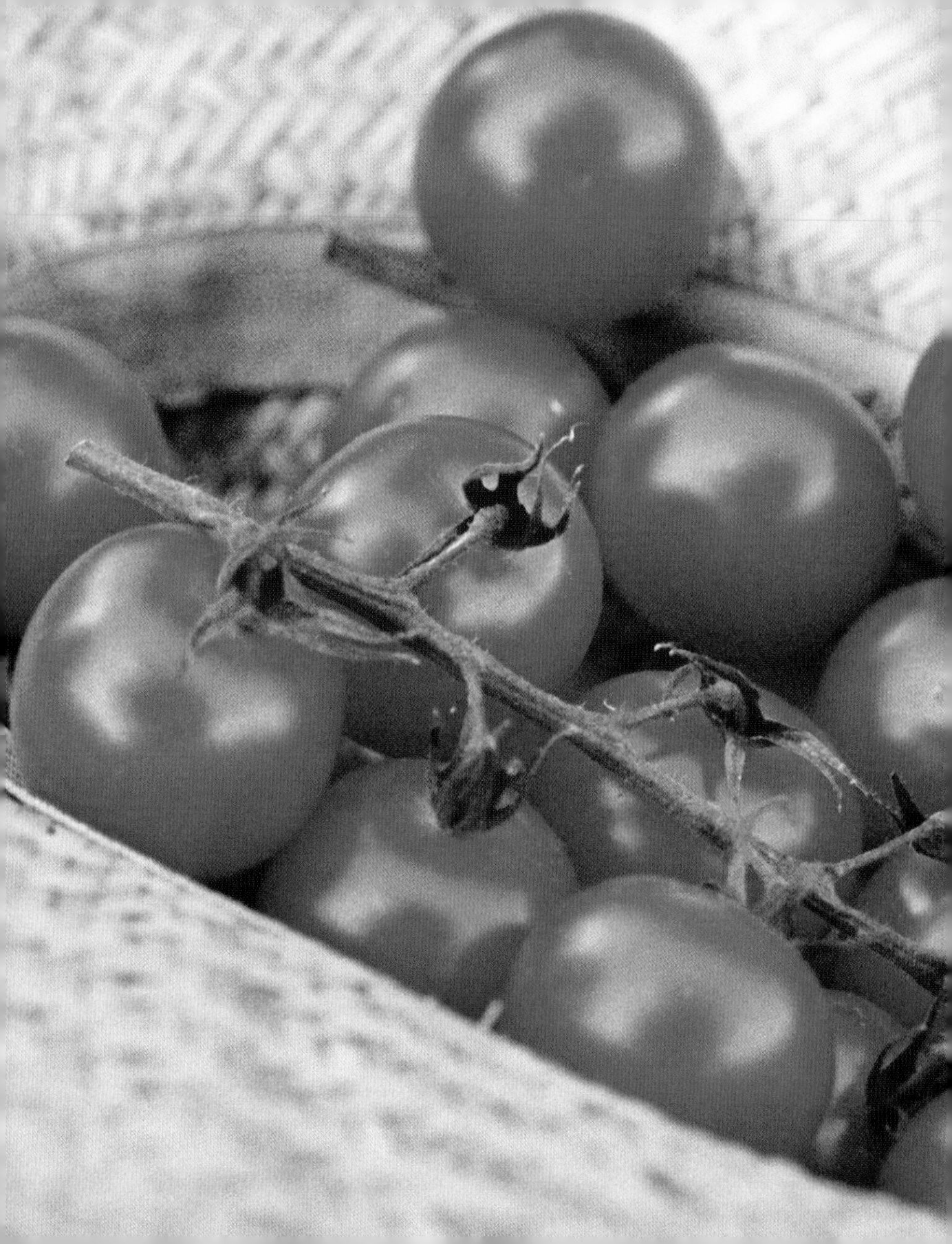

skin

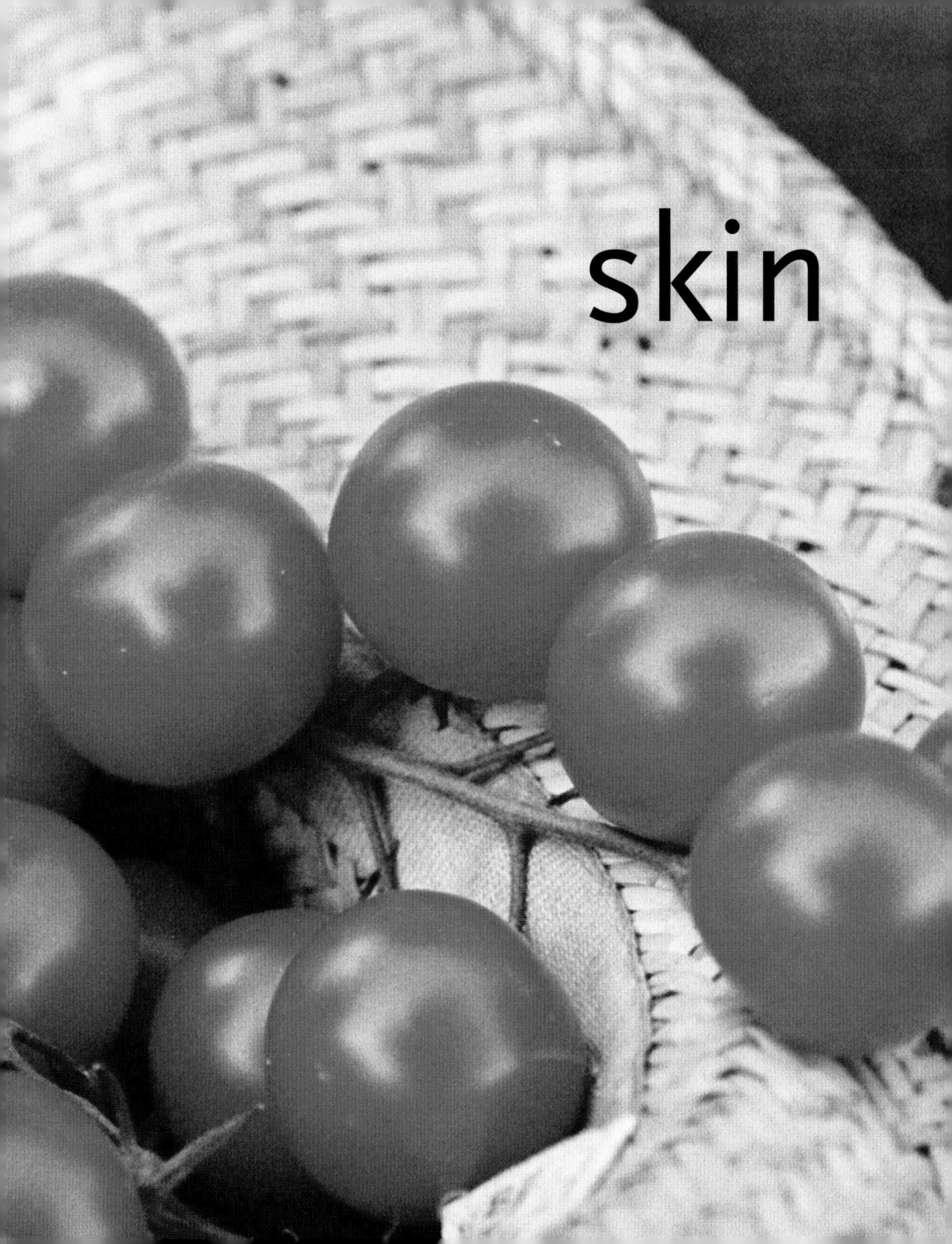

"Smooth as a baby's bottom" is a familiar phrase and certainly children as well as babies usually have silky soft, elastic, clear skin... if only the same applied to adults. It's not just the passage of time that changes our skin, but also the sun, cold, hormones and chemicals to which, children, by definition have been less exposed.

What we ingest into the body, and how well it is processed once it's in there, also affect the skin. How many children have come up in eczema when new foods are introduced into their diet? The skin can be seen as a barometer of what else is going on in the body – inflammation, stress and poor digestion can all show up as skin problems in children as well as in adults. So it is both outside and internal elements that determine the condition of your child's skin.

One of the most common skin problems in children is dry skin. This is hardly surprising given that the food intake of many children is devoid of the important fats needed to keep the skin well 'oiled' from the inside. The fats in nuts, seeds, avocados and fish are needed for (amongst other things) soft, healthy membranes in every skin cell (and elsewhere in the body). Without them, the skin becomes dry and scaly – crocodile legs! Having such oils in the skin cell membranes also means that they can, in effect, hold on to water better, so the cells remain nice and plump – more like fresh, soft, smooth apricots than crinkly dried ones.

The same oils can also be converted in the body to powerful chemicals that can reduce inflammation – essential in skin conditions such as eczema or psoriasis. So if your child suffers from eczema, including nuts, seeds and fish in their diet can help to calm the redness and 'moisturise' the skin from the inside. In many cases, a child's eczema is worsened by certain foods, for example dairy products, so you may find the information in Allergies (pages 98–9) useful.

Poor digestion, constipation and an imbalance in the micro-organisms in the digestive tract can affect the skin, triggering or exacerbating conditions such as acne and eczema, so the advice in Tummy (pages 60–1) may be particularly useful. If your child is hitting puberty and starting to get spotty, sticking to most of the wonderfoods throughout the book and steering clear of fried and sugary foods, and sugary drinks, can make a considerable difference.

Essential nutrients are needed to help the skin heal from the effects of eczema and acne, as well as from the typical cuts and grazes in childhood. Nutrients that are particularly important for skin healing are vitamin C, such as in strawberries and tomatoes, vitamin A (beta carotene) from carrots, and zinc in sunflower and sesame seeds.

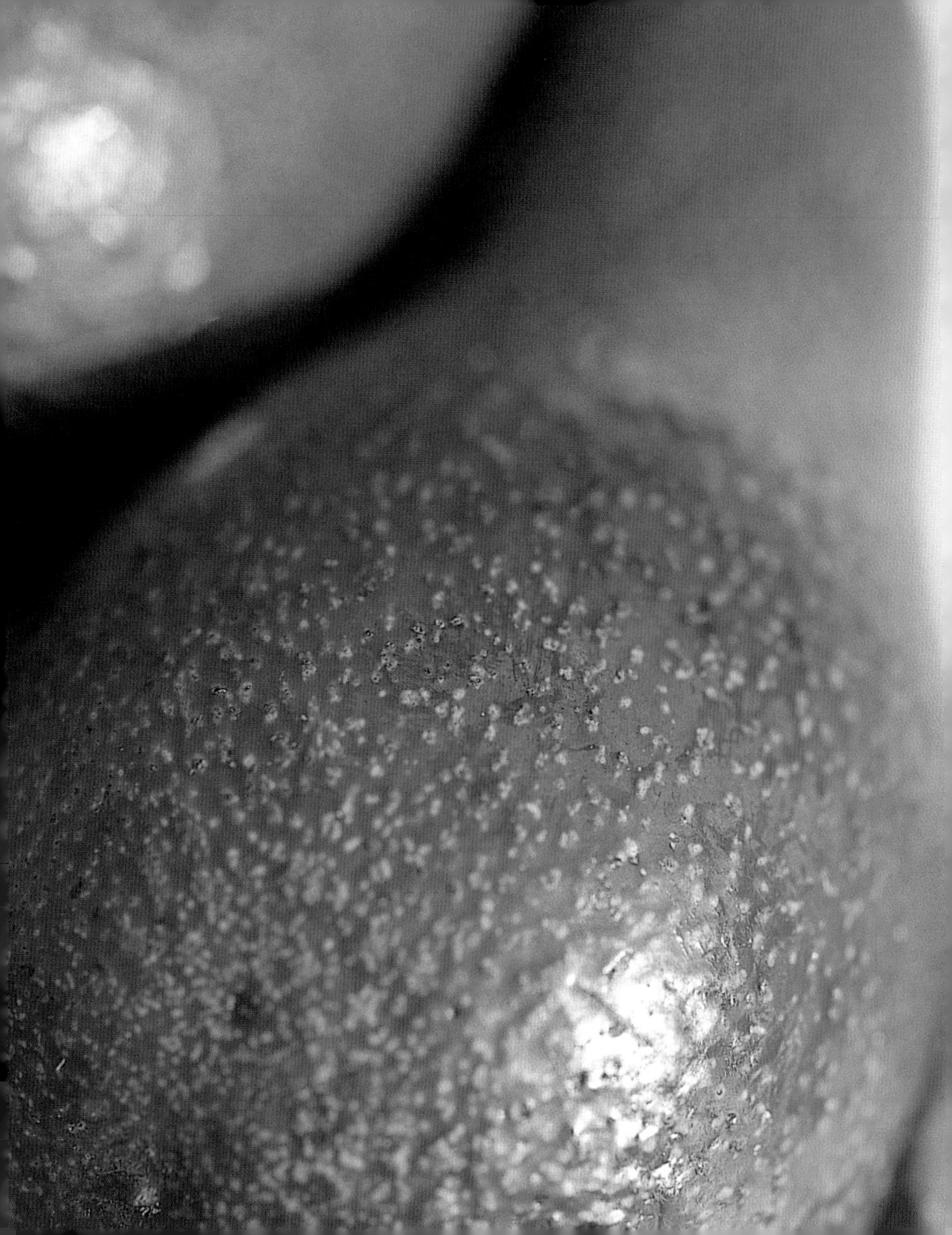

avocado

If your children are fans of so-called 'alligator pears', it is a real blessing to their health. Avocados are, when ripe, perfectly balanced. Neither acid nor alkaline, they are easily digestible and contain a wide range of beneficial oils, micronutrients and fibre. The rich oils in avocado are a blend of a little polyunsaturated (very desirable), saturated (not so desirable) and plenty of monounsaturated oleic acid, which is associated with good heart health. This fatty acid also keeps your child's skin soft and helps to guard it against oxidative damage, from sunburn for example. Avocados are a good source of fat-soluble vitamin E, which is needed to keep a child's skin elastic and smooth; it is particularly helpful in reducing scarring from wounds and the irritation of eczema. Another powerful antioxidant in avocados is lutein, which has a particular inclination towards protecting the eyes. Avocados also contain a cancer-protective chemical called beta-sitosterol. If your child isn't keen on the texture of avocado, try chopping and adding it to salads or mashing with other flavourings to make dips.

avocado dip & chips

THIS, ALONGSIDE CHICKPEA DIP (PAGE 89), MAKES A GREAT SUPPER FOR CHILDREN. THE DIP IS A GOOD SANDWICH FILLING FOR A PACKED LUNCH TOO.

FOR THE DIP
200g can ***tuna*** *in brine*
1 ripe ***avocado****, peeled*
2 tbsp cottage cheese
½ ***red pepper****, deseeded and finely diced*
juice of ¼ ***lemon***
1 tbsp olive oil
freshly ground black pepper
FOR THE 'CHIPS'
2 ***carrots****, peeled*
⅓ ***cucumber***
unsalted tortilla chips or root vegetable crisps

In a bowl, mash all the ingredients for the dip together with a fork until they are fairly smooth and well blended (young children can do this).

Cut the carrots and cucumber into batons and pile on to a plate with the tortilla chips or root crisps alongside. Serve with the dip.

ham & puy lentil salad

PUY LENTILS FROM FRANCE MAKE A GREAT SALAD AND THE CONTRASTING COLOURS IN THIS ONE ADD TO ITS APPEAL. COLD PRESSED SUNFLOWER OIL LENDS A NUTTY TOUCH – IF YOU CAN'T GET HOLD OF IT, USE OLIVE OIL INSTEAD, NOT COMMON SUPERMARKET SUNFLOWER OIL.

1 mugful of Puy ***lentils****, about 250g*
2 ***tomatoes***
2 spring ***onions****, trimmed and finely sliced*
2 thick slices of good quality cooked ham, chopped
6 ***basil*** *leaves, finely chopped*
2 tbsp cold pressed ***sunflower*** *(or olive) oil*
1 tbsp balsamic vinegar
freshly ground black pepper
pinch of sea salt
1 ripe ***avocado***

Wash the lentils and put them in a saucepan. Add water to cover generously and bring to the boil. Lower the heat and simmer until tender. This should take about 30 minutes.

While the lentils are cooking, add the tomatoes to the pan for a minute to loosen the skins, then remove with a slotted spoon and peel away the skins; set aside.

Taste the lentils to check that they are soft. Drain well, tip into a bowl and leave them to cool.

When the lentils are cooler, add the spring onions, ham, basil, oil, balsamic vinegar and seasoning. Toss to mix and leave for a couple of hours or so to allow the flavours to infuse (if you have time).

Just before serving, halve, stone and peel the avocado and dice the flesh. Roughly chop the peeled tomatoes. Toss the avocado and tomatoes through the salad and serve.

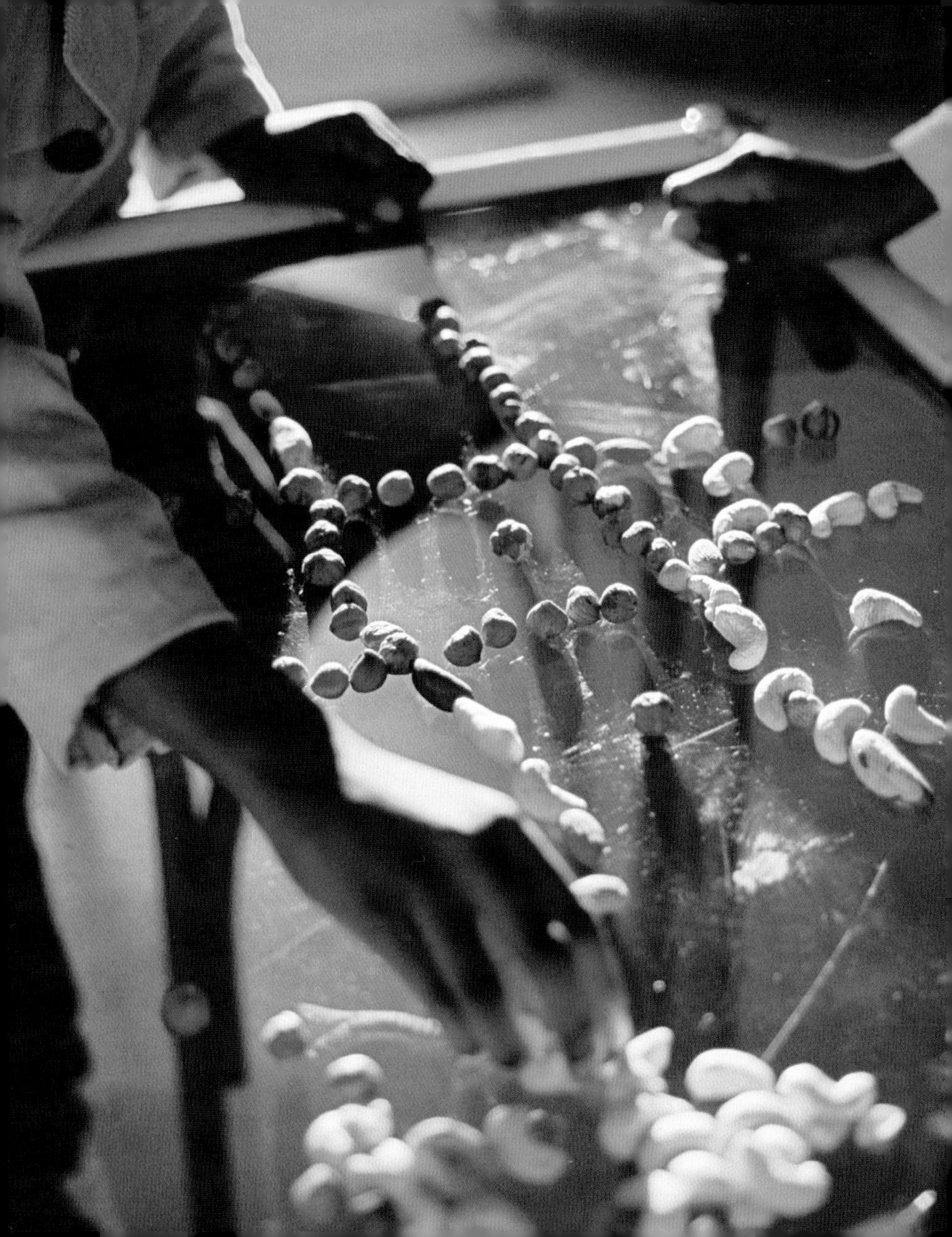

nuts

Giving nuts to your children is to hand them varied little packages of beneficial fats, proteins, vitamins and minerals, that is as long as they're not covered in chocolate, or salted. Offer them as a snack, in cereal, desserts, salads, etc., but not of course, if your child has an allergic reaction to them. Nuts are at least half fat, but it is of the 'good' variety, mainly mono-unsaturated (in almonds, like in olive oil) and polyunsaturated (the omega 3 fats in walnuts). So the fats are put to good use in your child's body, making for healthy skin, heart, brain and hormones. These fats come with protective antioxidants, like vitamin E, which keeps skin soft and supple and helps repair it after a cut. Nuts are a good source of protein, particularly for vegetarian or vegan children, while their fibre content helps keep the bowels healthy. They also provide vital nutrients such as calcium, magnesium, manganese and copper. Nuts are tough on digestion; soaking overnight makes them easier to break down, otherwise encourage your children to eat one nut at a time, chewing it to a paste before it goes down the hatch.

crunchy fish

THIS NUTTY CRUST WORKS WELL ON TOP OF ANY FISH, OR EVEN CHICKEN FILLETS. VARY IT BY USING BASIL OR CORIANDER INSTEAD OF THE PARSLEY.

4 chunky ***fish*** *fillets, such as cod or haddock*
FOR THE CRUST
4 tbsp ***almonds***
2 ***shallots****, peeled and quartered*
1 tbsp chopped ***parsley***
1 tsp Dijon mustard
juice of 1 ***lemon***

Preheat the oven to 180°C/Gas 4. To make the crust, use a pestle and mortar to grind the almonds, shallots, parsley, mustard and lemon juice together. (Young children could help here.)

Check the fish fillets for any small bones, then lay them in a baking dish. Smear the tops with the nutty mixture and spoon a little water round the fillets, just enough to thinly cover the bottom of the baking dish. This helps to keep the fish moist and makes it easier to remove from the dish.

Bake in the oven for 15–20 minutes until the fish is cooked through. Serve the crusted fillets with Spotty mash (page 81).

almond truffles

THESE SWEET TREATS ARE FUN AND EASY TO MAKE, EVEN WITH YOUNG CHILDREN.

250g ground ***almonds***
1 tbsp ***cocoa*** *powder*
5 tbsp runny ***honey***
FOR COATING
2 tbsp ***sesame seeds***
2 tbsp desiccated ***coconut***
2 tbsp ***hazelnuts****, finely chopped*

In a dry frying pan over a medium heat, stir the ground almonds until they are lightly coloured, being careful not to let them burn. Tip them out into a large bowl.

Add the cocoa powder and stir to blend in evenly, then gradually mix in the honey, a little at a time, stirring well to make a smooth, thick truffle mixture. (It's easier to mix in if you gently warm the honey to make it more liquid, but I don't usually bother dirtying another pan!)

Using your hands (and the children's), take little pieces and roll into small balls – no more than 2.5cm in diameter, as they're very rich.

Leave some truffles plain. Roll others in sesame seeds, coconut or chopped hazelnuts to coat all over. Place on a tray lined with baking paper and chill until ready to eat.

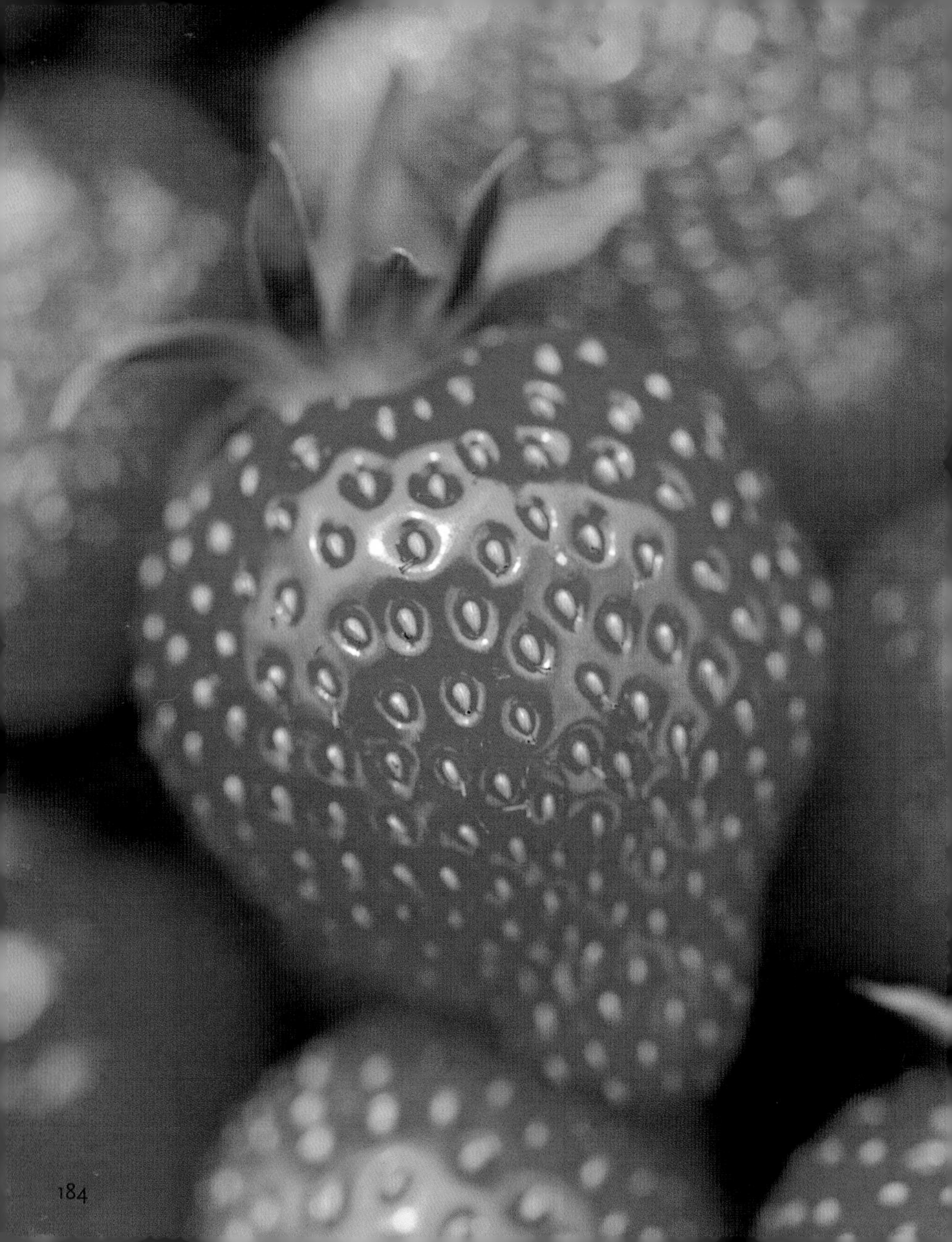

strawberry

The most popular of all berries, the strawberry is particularly appealing in taste and 'cuteness' to children. Indeed, many child-orientated products are branded strawberry-flavoured to broaden their appeal... anything from toothpaste to sweets. Strawberries are a wonderfully rich source of vitamin C, one of the skin's favourite nutrients. It is essential for building collagen, or 'cellular glue', which holds us all together. Healthy skin growth and repair (from cuts, spots and eczema scratches) depend on decent levels of vitamin C, as well as nutrients like zinc, which is found in strawberries too. Both also contribute to healthy defences in your child and a good stress response. Just three or four strawberries provide a child's daily need of vitamin C. These sweet berries owe their appealing colour at least in part to powerful antioxidant substances called anthocyanins, which help protect not only the skin but all of the body's tissues from oxidant damage. They also help reduce inflammation, which is useful in asthma and eczema. Other antioxidants, ellagitannins, are linked to lower risks of cancer.

grilled chicken & strawberry salsa

THIS SALSA IS PARTICULARLY GOOD IN SUMMER WHEN STRAWBERRIES ARE AT THEIR PEAK AND YOU'VE GOT FRESH CHICKEN COOKING ON A BARBECUE.

8 ***chicken*** *thighs (or drumsticks or breast fillets if you like)*
FOR THE SALSA
250g ***strawberries****, hulled*
1 tbsp sweet chilli sauce
juice of 1/2 ***lime***
1 tbsp chopped ***mint***

Preheat the grill to high (or light the barbecue and wait until the coals burn white). Grill the chicken (or barbecue) for 2–3 minutes on each side, then turn down the grill to a low-medium heat (or move the chicken to a cooler part of the barbecue). Cook, turning occasionally, for a further 20 minutes, or until the chicken thighs are cooked through. To test, pierce the thickest part with a knife or skewer – the juices should run clear.

Meanwhile, for the salsa, chop the strawberries into small pieces and place in a bowl with the chilli sauce, lime and mint. Toss to mix.

Serve the cooked chicken with the strawberry salsa and side dishes such as Sesame beans (page 137) and Squish squash (page 32).

strawbs in skirts

THESE ARE A GREAT TREAT FOR TEA OR A LIGHT DESSERT. MAKE SURE THE STRAWBERRIES ARE NICE AND RIPE.

500g ***strawberries****, with hulls*
200g dark ***chocolate****, broken into pieces*
100g white chocolate, broken into pieces

Wipe the strawberries with damp kitchen paper to clean them. Line a tray with greaseproof paper.

Put the two types of chocolate into separate, heatproof bowls and rest them over small pans of boiling water, making sure the base of the bowls isn't in contact with the water. Leave until the chocolate has melted, stirring occasionally.

Holding it by the hull, partially dip each strawberry into one of the bowls of melted chocolate to coat the bottom half, allow excess chocolate to drip off, then lay on the paper-lined tray. Coat half the strawberries with white and half with dark chocolate, or try coating some half white, half dark. (Young children can have a go at this if you take the bowls off the pans and make sure they are careful.)

Leave the tray of strawberries in a cool place for at least 2 hours until the chocolate has set.

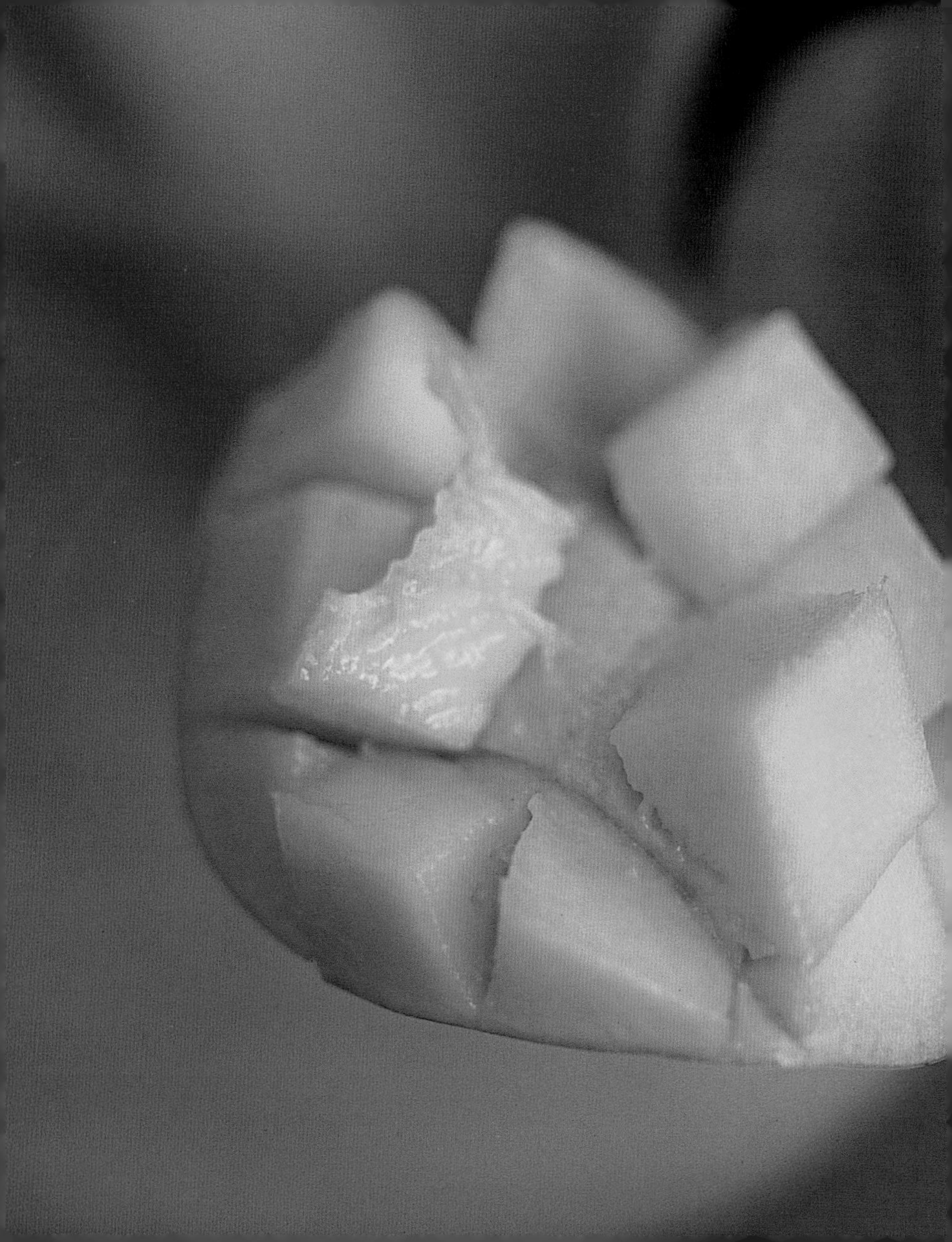

mango

Mangoes were such a treat when I was a child (as they still are) and there was only one way to enjoy them: strip down to my knickers, sit at the table and squish the flesh all inside its skin before biting a hole, sucking out the juice (licking the rest off the table) and scraping the stone until it was dry and my teeth were riddled with mango 'hair'. Little did I know then what goodness I was tucking into, especially as I grew up in the Arabian Gulf where my skin was exposed to strong sunshine. As their bright orange colour suggests, mangoes are loaded with beta carotene, an antioxidant that helps protect the skin from the elements. It is also useful for keeping lungs, eyes and the lining of the gut healthy. Other powerful antioxidants in mangoes are vitamins C and E (both needed for unblemished skin), as well as phenols such as quercetin. Mangoes are also a very good source of dietary fibre, which helps to eliminate wastes effectively from the body and can relieve constipation. They also contain small amounts of the full spectrum of other vitamins and minerals, making them a true wonderfood.

mango hedgehog

MANGOES ARE SO PRECIOUS – ESPECIALLY WHEN YOU BUY THEM ANYWHERE THEY'RE NOT GROWN – IT SEEMS WRONG TO ADULTERATE THEM. HERE'S A WAY OF CUTTING THEM UP TO MAKE THEM MORE FUN FOR CHILDREN.

1 ***mango*** *per child*

Holding the mango upright, slice down each side from top to bottom, close to the stone, so you have two 'almost halfs' with a middle slice clinging to the stone.

Cut across the flesh of each mango 'half' in parallel lines – carefully so as not to cut through the skin. Now cut across these lines in the same way, so you have criss-crossed flesh with the skin perfectly intact.

Turn the skin in on itself so you have a mound of 'spikes' for the children to eat (they can do this themselves). Just let them slurp and nibble at the other slice surrounding the stone.

mango & sweet potato salad

THIS SALAD IS GREAT WITH STICKY CHICKEN (PAGE 153) OR DUSTED DRUMSTICKS (PAGE 72). IT CAN EVEN MAKE A SOPHISTICATED ADDITION TO A LUNCHBOX.

1 small ***sweet potato****, peeled*
1 ***mango***
1 ***garlic*** *clove, peeled and crushed*
juice of 1 ***lime***
1 tsp Thai fish sauce (or tamari)
1 tbsp ***sesame*** *oil*
1 tbsp chopped ***coriander***

Cut the sweet potato into chunks, put into in a saucepan, add water to cover and bring to the boil. Cook for about 7 minutes until tender but not mushy. Drain and set aside to cool.

Peel and slice the mango off the stone and place in a large bowl. Add the garlic, lime juice, fish sauce, sesame oil and chopped coriander and toss to mix (small children can do this).

When it is cool, add the sweet potato to the salad, toss again, then it's ready.

sunflower & sesame seeds

Sunflowers are so stunning, it's hardly surprising that they yield such goodness in the form of their seeds, which, in themselves, are not much to look at. Similarly, tiny sesame seeds pack a robust nutritional punch for children. Both seeds and their oils are excellent sources of essential fats, especially the omega 6 variety needed for healthy skin, hormone balance and to combat inflammation (useful in conditions like asthma and eczema). Omega 6s are also linked to reducing hyperactivity. The seeds contain another skin-friendly nutrient, vitamin E, which helps keep the skin soft and supple. The zinc in both seeds is useful for the creation of new skin cells, in everyday growth but also repair; it's crucial to help children through growth spurts and for good defences against infections. Both seeds are rich in the antioxidant, cancer-protective mineral selenium, as well as calcium and magnesium. These latter two are used to build healthy bones and to help muscles relax and contract properly. This doesn't just mean the muscles in your children's arms and legs but also internal muscles, such as in the heart.

seedy snack

THIS IS A GREAT SNACK FOR CHILDREN THAT CAN ALSO BE SPRINKLED ON TO COOKED VEG OR RICE. YOU CAN MAKE UP A BIG BATCH IN ADVANCE AND STORE IT IN AN AIRTIGHT CONTAINER.

3 tbsp ***sunflower seeds***
3 tbsp ***pumpkin seeds***
2 tbsp ***sesame seeds***
1 tbsp tamari (or soy sauce)

Preheat the oven to 170°C/Gas 3. Line a baking tray with baking paper. Mix all the seeds together in a bowl with the tamari so they are well coated, then spread them out on the baking tray. (Children can do this.)

Put the tray in the oven and toast the seeds for 15 minutes, shaking or stirring them a couple of times to ensure they colour evenly.

Leave the toasted seeds to cool before giving them to children or storing away.

monster chomp cereal

THIS IS A SWEET, TOASTED GRANOLA THAT MAKES A GREAT ALTERNATIVE TO THE PROCESSED, OVER-SWEETENED BREAKFAST CEREALS MARKETED TO CHILDREN. YOU COULD USE ANY DRIED FRUIT OR OTHER PUFFED GRAINS AVAILABLE FROM A HEALTH FOOD SHOP.

200g porridge ***oats***
200g ***rye*** *flakes*
3 tbsp ***sunflower seeds***
2 tbsp ***pumpkin seeds***
2 tbsp ***sesame seeds***
2 tbsp ***almonds*** *or* ***hazelnuts****, roughly broken*
8 tbsp ***honey***
8 tbsp ***coconut*** *oil or olive oil*
2 tsp vanilla extract
3 tbsp ***raisins***
8 dried ***apricots****, finely chopped*
50g puffed ***quinoa***

Preheat the oven to 160°C/Gas 2½. Line a large shallow baking tin (or two smaller ones) with greaseproof paper. In a large bowl, mix together the oats, rye, seeds and nuts.

Put the honey, oil and vanilla extract in a small saucepan and heat gently – just enough to melt it all together. Pour on to the cereal mixture and stir it through well.

Spread the mixture out in the lined baking tin(s) and bake for about 25 minutes, shaking it up halfway through and lowering the heat a little if it appears to be colouring too quickly.

Leave the toasted cereal to cool, then mix in the dried fruit and puffed quinoa. Store in an airtight container. Serve the children a bowlful for breakfast with milk or soya milk.

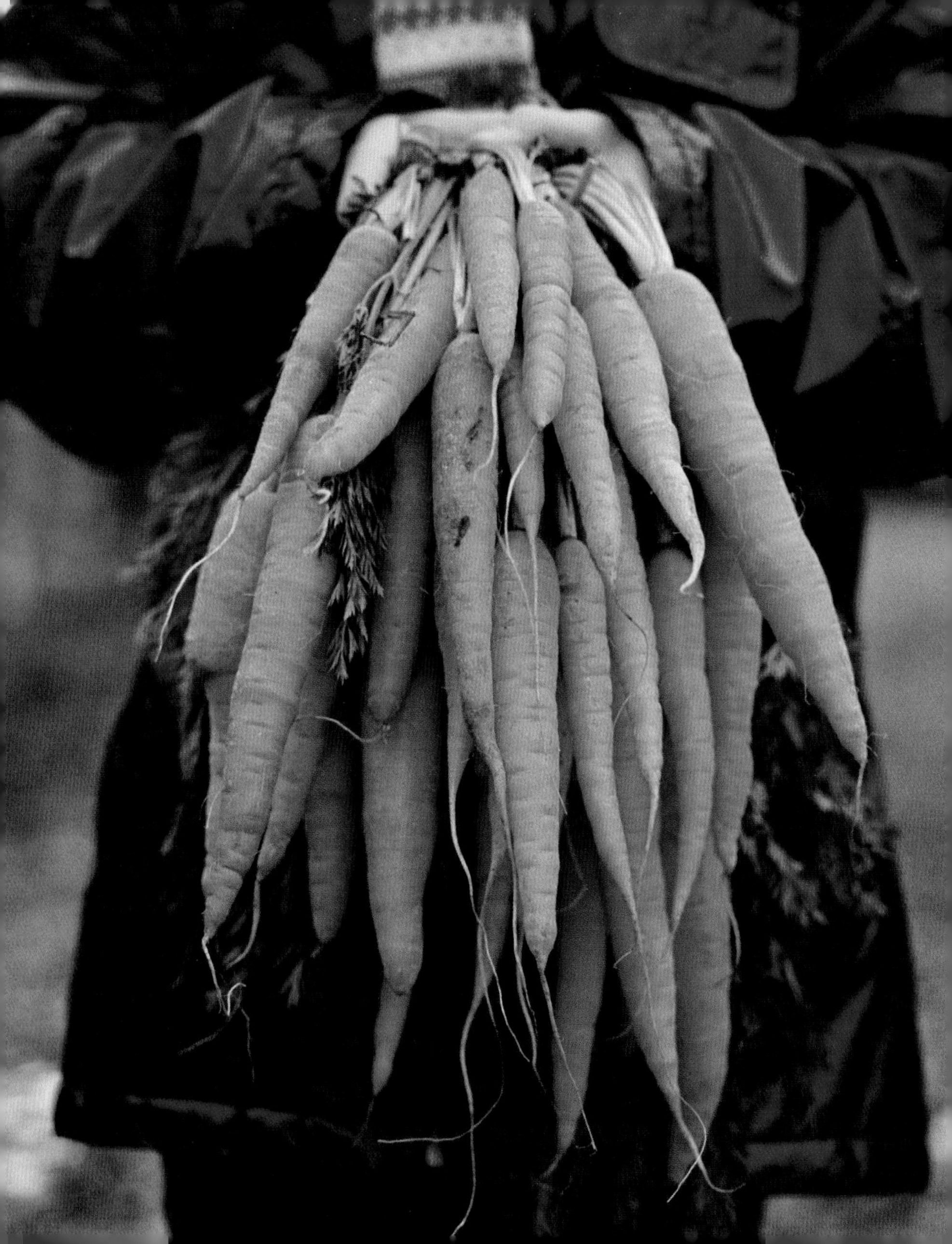

carrot

"*Nyaaaah. Wassup doc?*" Bugs Bunny mechanically chomping through a carrot comes to mind whenever I'm faced with a carrot baton (in selected company, I succumb and mimic him)! These humble vegetable sticks are often one of a baby's first solid foods and a very good one too. Carrots' best known value of helping us see well at night is grounded in scientific fact. Their rich beta carotene content can be converted in the body into vitamin A and put to good use in not only children's eyes, but also their skin, immune systems, lungs and digestive tracts. The vitamin A is used to make rhodopsin in the eye, which is needed for seeing in the dark. It also helps lung health, important in children with asthma and for warding off chest infections. Another benefit for the skin provided by carrots is silica. Carrots' sweetness comes from their relatively high sugar content, which partly accounts for their popularity with children. They are also packed with fibre that, particularly when cooked, is easily digested. This fibre, together with the beta carotene, makes them soothing for tummy problems.

carrot ribbon salad

PART OF THE FUN HERE IS THE RIBBON SHAPED CARROTS. THE SALAD GOES WELL WITH ANY FISH OR CHICKEN DISH, SUCH AS FISH IN SLEEPING BAGS (PAGE 77), OR IN A PACKED LUNCH.

3 ***carrots****, peeled*
juice of 1 ***orange***
2 tbsp ***sesame*** *oil*
2 tsp tamari (or soy sauce)
2 tbsp ***pumpkin seeds***

Using a swivel potato peeler, slice the carrots thinly lengthways to make long ribbons.

Put the carrots into a bowl, add the orange juice, sesame oil and tamari and toss the carrot ribbons so they are well coated (small children can do this). Add the pumpkin seeds and toss again.

Serve the salad as a side dish or as part of a packed lunch.

sweet minty carrots

THE SWEETNESS OF THE CARROTS AND THE FAMILIAR FLAVOUR OF MINT MAKE THIS VEGETABLE SIDE DISH A HIT WITH MOST CHILDREN. IT GOES WELL WITH ANY MAIN COURSE SUCH AS DUSTED DRUMSTICKS (PAGE 72) OR LENTIL STACKS (PAGE 95).

3 ***carrots****, peeled*
3–4 tbsp water
1 tsp runny **honey**
1 tbsp olive oil
1 tsp finely chopped **mint**

Thinly slice the carrots on the diagonal, or whichever way you like (though thin slices will cook more quickly).

Put the carrot slices in a wok or large saucepan with the water and honey and toss them around over a medium-high heat for 3–4 minutes.

Add the olive oil and toss the carrots for another minute before adding the chopped mint. Toss over the heat for a final minute, then serve.

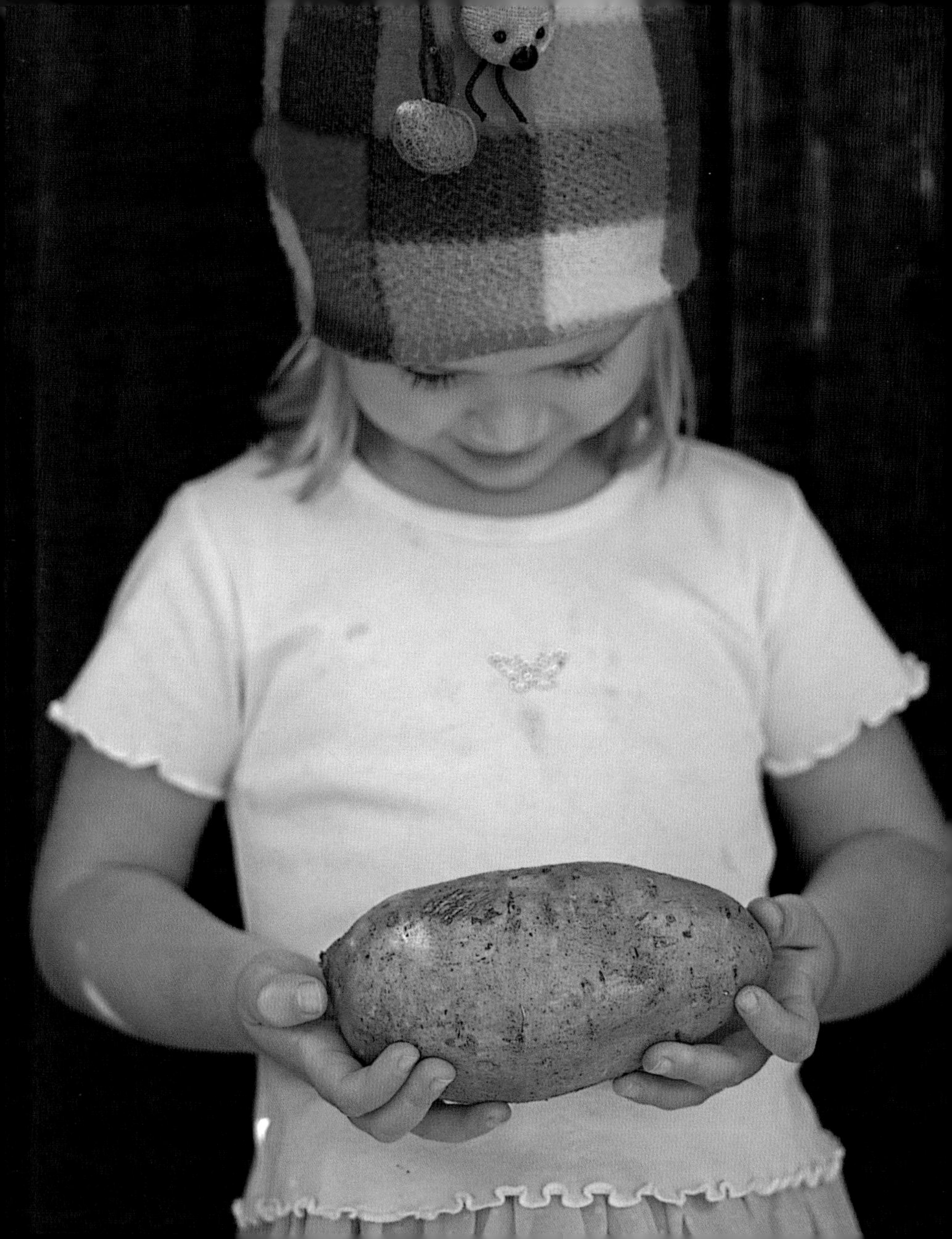

sweet potato

This West Indian native come in many shapes and colours, but the sweetest and most nutritious are the orange-fleshed, dusty pink-skinned sweet potatoes. When roasted slowly, their sweetness intensifies, as they almost caramelise – tempting most children. Beneficially, sweet potatoes release their energy gently rather than giving a rapid 'high'. They are also easily digested and their high fibre content keeps the guts moving well, which is relevant for spotty teenagers. The bright orange colour not only looks appealing but also hints at the high levels of beta carotene. This plant form of vitamin A is very much linked to healthy skin. It is needed for skin cells to regenerate, which they do constantly; it helps healing after a cut, graze, spot or eczema has damaged the skin; it's also important for the health of 'internal skin' that lines the digestive system and lungs, therefore useful for a child with sensitive digestion or a tendency to coughs. The beta carotene, along with vitamin C, another valuable antioxidant in sweet potatoes, gives them further defence-boosting and anti-inflammatory properties.

gobble pie

THIS LIGHTER, MORE NUTRIENT-PACKED VERSION OF A TRADITIONAL MEAT AND POTATO PIE IS A GREAT FAMILY MEAL. FOR A VEGETARIAN ALTERNATIVE, REPLACE THE TURKEY WITH A COUPLE OF CANS OF LENTILS OR BEANS.

500g sweet potatoes *(2 large ones), peeled and cubed*
2–3 ***garlic*** *cloves, peeled*
1 large ***onion****, peeled and chopped*
2–3 tbsp olive oil
1 ***carrot****, peeled and finely chopped*
1 celery stick, finely chopped
400g ***turkey*** *mince*
2 tsp tamari (or soy sauce)
2 tsp Worcestershire sauce
1 bay leaf
1 tbsp ***tomato*** *purée*
400g can chopped ***tomatoes***
150ml water
2 tbsp chopped ***parsley***
2 tbsp ***sesame seeds***

Preheat the oven to 190°C/Gas 5. Put the sweet potato cubes in a pan with 1–2 garlic cloves, add water to cover and bring to the boil. Cover and simmer until tender. Crush the other garlic clove.

Meanwhile, in a large pan, soften the onion in 1 tbsp olive oil over a medium heat for 5 minutes. Add the carrot, celery, crushed garlic and turkey mince and stir until the meat is evenly coloured. Stir in the tamari, Worcestershire sauce, bay leaf, tomato purée, tomatoes, water and parsley. Partially cover the pan and simmer for 10 minutes.

When the sweet potatoes are cooked, drain them well and mash together with the garlic and 1–2 tbsp olive oil.

Tip the turkey mixture into a baking dish, pouring off some of the liquid if it is too watery and discarding the bay leaf. Cover it evenly with the mashed sweet potato and sprinkle the sesame seeds on top. Bake for 20–30 minutes, or until the potato is just starting to brown. Serve with a plain steamed green vegetable, such as broccoli.

bright bubble & squeak

THIS IS A DELICIOUS TWIST ON THE TRADITIONAL GREEN CABBAGE AND POTATO VERSION. IT GOES WELL WITH ANY MEAT OR FISH MAIN COURSE, SUCH AS BAKED PORK WITH APPLES (PAGE 64).

2 ***sweet potatoes****, peeled and diced*
wedge of red ***cabbage****, finely shredded*
1 leek, trimmed and very finely chopped
1 tbsp olive oil

Put the sweet potato cubes in a saucepan, add water to cover generously and bring to the boil. Cook for about 7 minutes until soft, adding the cabbage to the pan for the last minute. Drain well, then tip both vegetables into a bowl, add the leek and mash them all together.

Heat the olive oil in a frying pan. Add the sweet potato mixture – either as one big 'cake' or shaped into smaller patties. Flatten slightly with a fish slice and fry for 4 or 5 minutes on each side. Serve straight away.

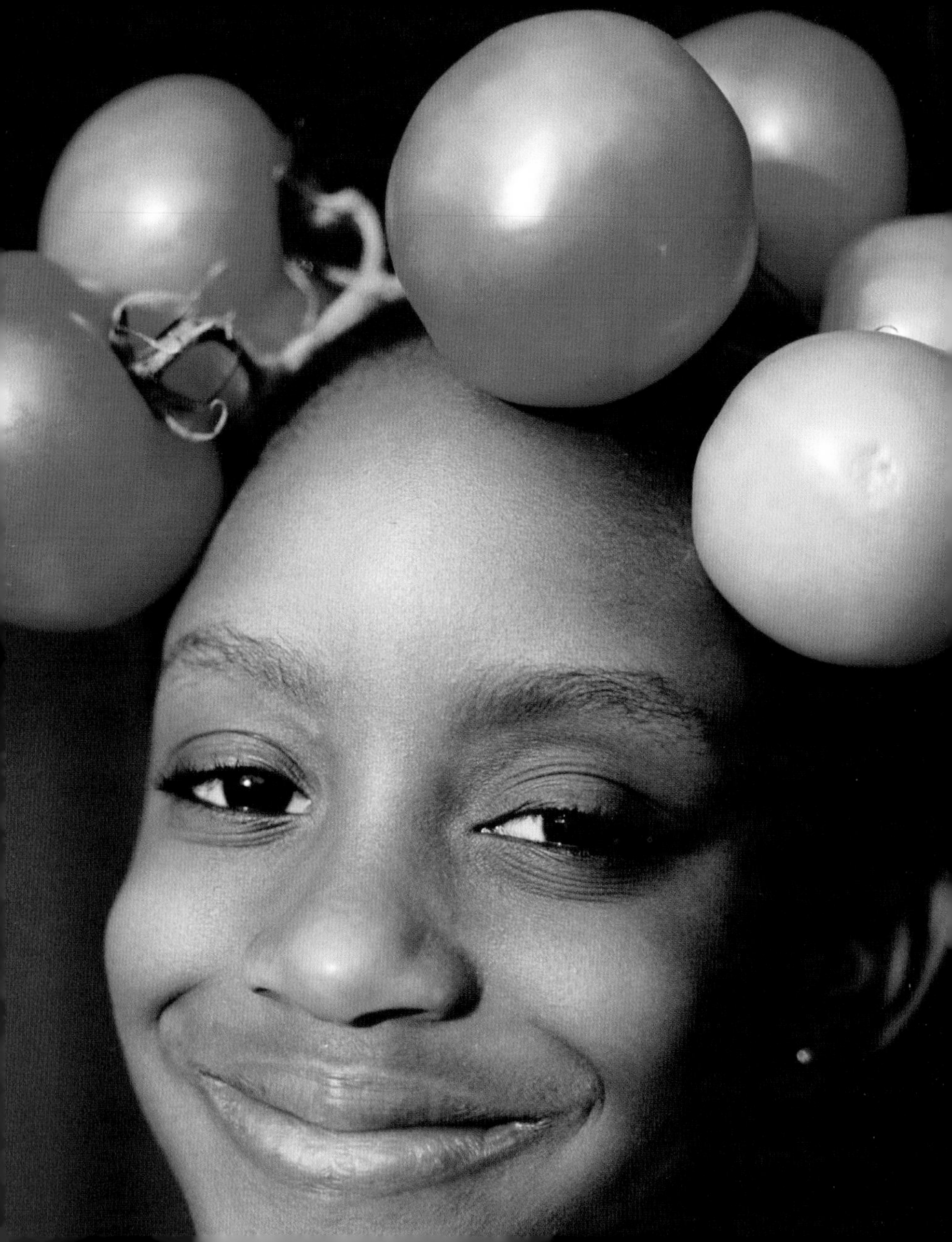

tomato

My earliest memory of tomatoes is the gnarled, misshapen ones, which we would squish on to bread, dip in olive oil and devour in my grandmother's kitchen in Malta. It is hard to find such delicious tomatoes these days, but worth the hunt. Tomatoes are packed with goodness; their best known assets are antioxidant carotenoids such as lycopene, which contribute to their red colour and safeguarding properties. Lycopene has been shown to protect the skin and eyes from sun damage and to help reduce the risk of cancer. Tomatoes are a great source of vitamin C – used by your child's body to build and repair skin, boost immunity, mount a stress response and more. Tomatoes have not always been so highly rated – their Latin name, *Lycopersicon*, means 'wolf peach', apparently referring to their supposed harmful properties. Anecdotal evidence suggests that some children with conditions such as eczema, hives and arthritis, benefit from avoiding the 'nightshade' family of vegetables, which includes tomatoes. Otherwise tomatoes dose your children up with amazing goodness.

big tomato sandwich

THIS IS ONE OF MY FAVOURITE SANDWICH FILLINGS – TANGY TOMATOES AND CREAMY FETA, ALL OFFSET WITH GARLICKY HOUMMOUS... PERHAPS NOT THE MOST SOCIAL PACKED LUNCH IN THE SCHOOL CANTEEN, BUT DELICIOUS NONETHELESS!

8 slices ***rye*** *bread*
4 tsp hoummous
4 medium, ripe ***tomatoes****, sliced*
100g feta cheese, crumbled
freshly ground black pepper

Spread the slices of rye bread with hoummous (a tasty alternative to butter). Lay the tomatoes on top of four of the slices, then pile on the feta. Season with pepper and top with the other four slices of bread. Serve at once or wrap up and pack into lunchboxes.

meatballs in tomato sauce

THIS, OR SOMETHING APPROXIMATING IT, TAKES ME BACK TO MY GRANDMOTHER'S COMFORTING, BLUE KITCHEN IN MALTA. WE USED TO HAVE SPAGHETTI WITH OUR MEATBALLS BUT BROWN RICE IS GOOD TOO, DUSTED WITH MORE PARMESAN.

FOR THE MEATBALLS
500g very lean beef mince
1 ***garlic*** *clove, peeled and finely chopped*
2 tbsp freshly grated Parmesan cheese
1 ***egg****, beaten*
handful of ***parsley****, very finely chopped*
pinch of sea salt (optional)
freshly ground black pepper
flour, to dust
2 tbsp olive oil, for frying
FOR THE SAUCE
1 ***onion****, peeled and finely chopped*
2 ***garlic*** *cloves, peeled and crushed*
1 celery stick, very finely chopped
2 x 400g cans chopped ***tomatoes***
2 tbsp ***tomato*** *purée*
splash of ***apple*** *juice*
1 bay leaf
100g ***peas*** *(frozen is fine)*

To make the meatballs, put the minced beef in a large bowl and add the garlic, Parmesan, egg, parsley and seasoning. Gently mix the ingredients together using your hands until evenly combined.

Dust your surface with flour (or buckwheat flour if avoiding wheat). Shape meatballs, the size of a golf ball, with your hands and roll on the surface to dust with flour. (Small children can do this.)

Heat the olive oil in a large, wide saucepan. Lower the heat and brown the meatballs in batches, turning them to colour on all sides. Remove with a slotted spoon and drain on kitchen paper.

For the sauce, add the onion, garlic and celery to the same pan and cook gently for 10 minutes, or until the onion is soft. Stir in the tomatoes and mush them with the spoon. Add the tomato purée, apple juice and bay leaf and bring to a simmer. Lower the meatballs into the sauce and leave it all to simmer, covered, for at least half an hour, adding the peas for the last 5–10 minutes.

Serve piled on to portions of rice or pasta.

stuffed tomatoes

IF YOUR CHILD IS ALLERGIC TO – OR DOESN'T LIKE – FISH, JUST SUBSTITUTE THE SARDINES WITH FETA OR MOZZARELLA CHEESE.

8 medium, ripe ***tomatoes***
125g canned ***sardines****, drained*
8 black olives, pitted and chopped
juice of ½ ***lemon***
1 tbsp sweet chilli sauce
1 tbsp finely chopped ***parsley***
1 tsp olive oil

Preheat the oven to 200°C/Gas 6. Slice the tops off the tomatoes and carefully scoop out the flesh and seeds, spooning the flesh into a bowl.

Add the sardines, olives, lemon juice, chilli sauce and chopped parsley to the tomato flesh and mash together roughly, using a fork. (Small children can do this.)

Stuff the tomatoes with the mash, replace the tops and put them on an oiled baking tray. Drizzle a little olive oil over them and bake the tomatoes in the oven for 10–15 minutes until they just begin to soften. Serve them with warm brown rolls.

speedy pizzas

THIS IS REALLY A FANCY VERSION OF CHEESE ON TOAST THAT CHILDREN CAN EASILY ASSEMBLE THEMSELVES.

3 ripe ***tomatoes***
1 tbsp pesto
8 slices wholemeal bread, lightly toasted
FOR THE TOPPINGS
choose from:
canned ***tuna****, flaked*
slices of ham, cubed
smoked ***tofu****, cubed*
olives, pitted
chestnut ***mushrooms****, finely sliced*
mozzarella, finely cubed (or firm cheese, grated)

Preheat the oven to 190°C/Gas 5. Line a baking tray with greaseproof paper. Dip the tomatoes in a small pan of boiling water for a minute to loosen the skins, then remove and peel. Finely chop the flesh and mix with the pesto in a small bowl.

Spread the tomato pesto on the slices of toast and get each child to top their two slices with any of the other ingredients they fancy.

Lay the slices of toast on the baking tray and bake them in the oven for about 7–10 minutes, until any cheese is bubbling.

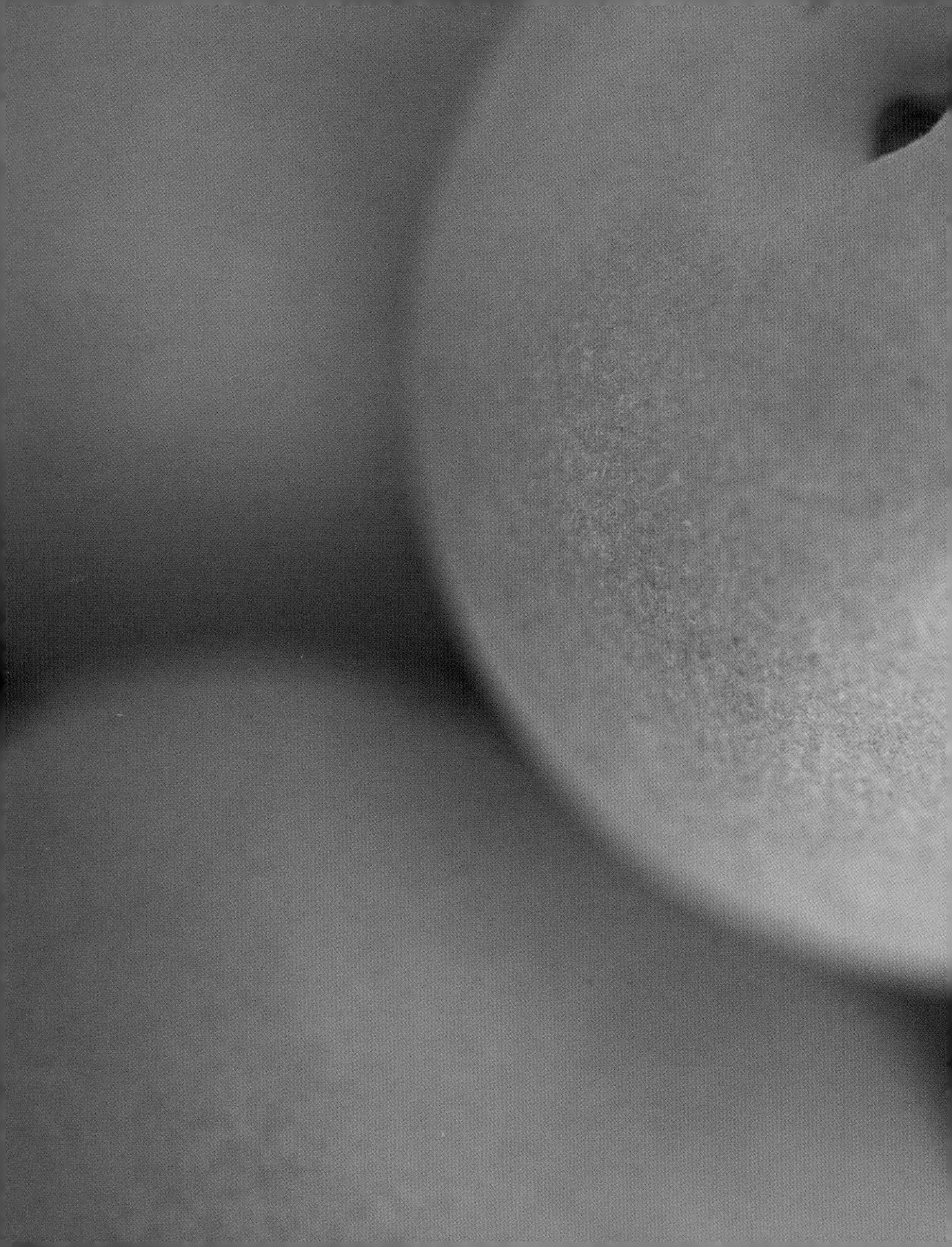

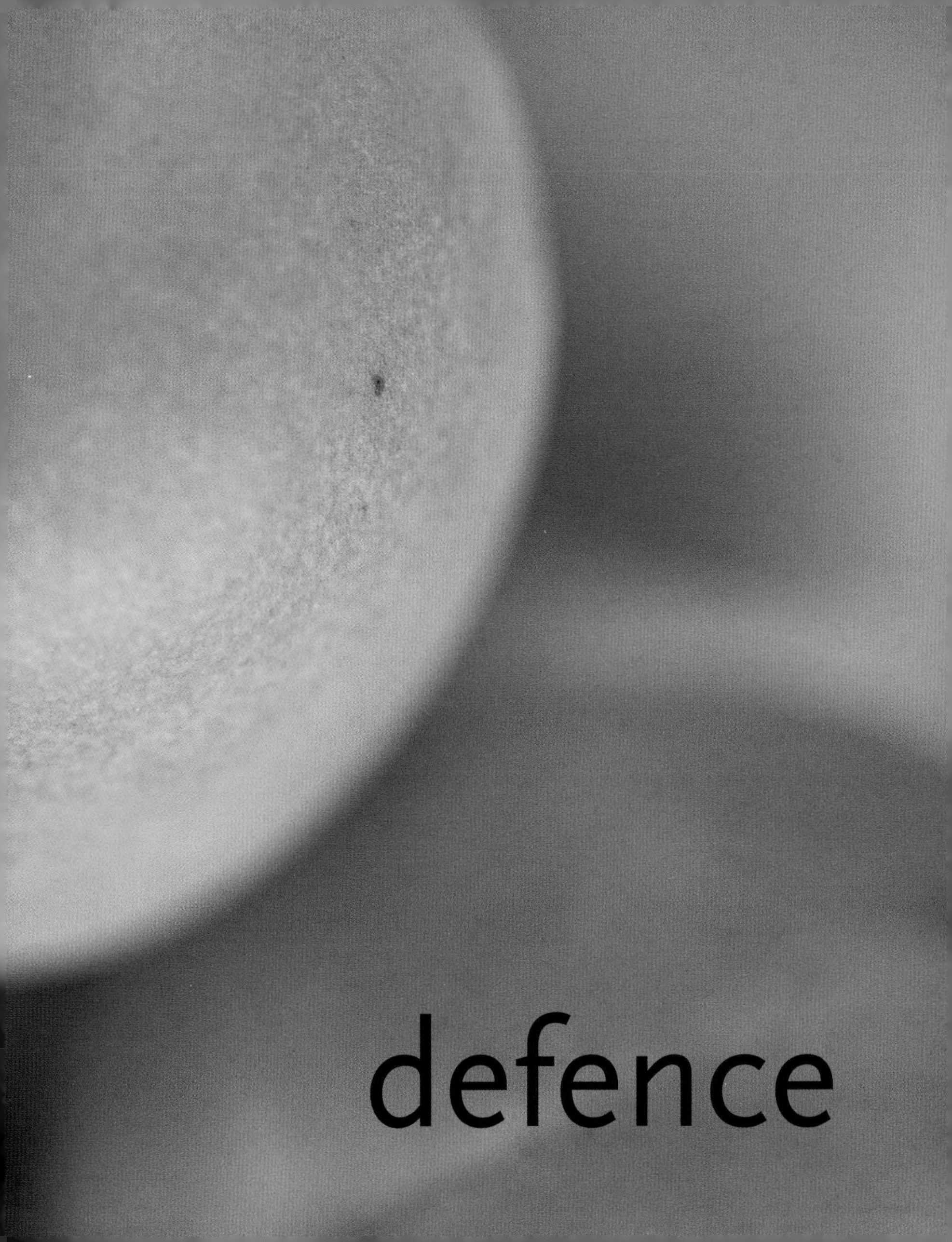
defence

You'll probably recognise many of the foods in this chapter as ones that are renowned for giving the body a good boost when it's fighting off something. Children who have a healthy diet, which includes foods in this section, are less likely to succumb to an illness. And when they are unwell, it's worth calling on these foods to give their immunity a good kick. Traditional remedies, such as lemons for a cold, are now known to stand up to scientific scrutiny, owing to their content of vitamin C and other powerful antioxidant nutrients. Similarly kiwis, pomegranates and other fruits are now confirming their old-fashioned reputations for harbouring goodness. While certain mushrooms, which have been renowned in Japan for centuries as enhancing the body's defences, are now available across the world and are getting scientific endorsement for their powers.

Your child's immune system is continually developing. From their first breath, babies are building up the resources to handle 'foreign invaders' that come their way. And as children grow, their systems are constantly evolving in order to combat illness. The immune system is extraordinarily complex and consists of a range of organs, sites and cells across the body. It is designed to deal with viruses, bacteria, parasites, allergy-triggers, debris around cuts and grazes, and some chemicals. All the places where your child's 'insides' open up to the outside world, there are mechanisms in place to fend off potential disease. For example, there are immune cells lining the respiratory passages and gut, and protective chemicals on the skin and in tears. Then inside the body itself, more cells lie in wait or actively patrol to pounce on would-be invaders and dangerously mutating cells that could turn cancerous.

The key to defending your child's body is not simply to try to avoid exposure to harmful organisms, which isn't really possible anyway. But it is to make sure he or she is as healthy as possible all of the time so that when a bug passes, it is less likely to be able to have an effect. It's no coincidence that in a class of children some will fall ill to a passing infection while others remain well. If a bug lands in weakened territory, it is more likely to take a steadfast hold. Diet is not the only factor in determining the strength of the immune system – tiredness and stress undermine the body's ability to fend off illness.

Incorporate the wonderfoods in this chapter as regular features in your child's diet and he or she will be exposed to a range of foods that are not only tasty and versatile, but also known to contribute to a heightened immune system. When potential illness comes its way, your child's immune system will be ready and alert to defend his or her body. It also means that your child is less likely to develop or fall prey to the symptoms of allergies.

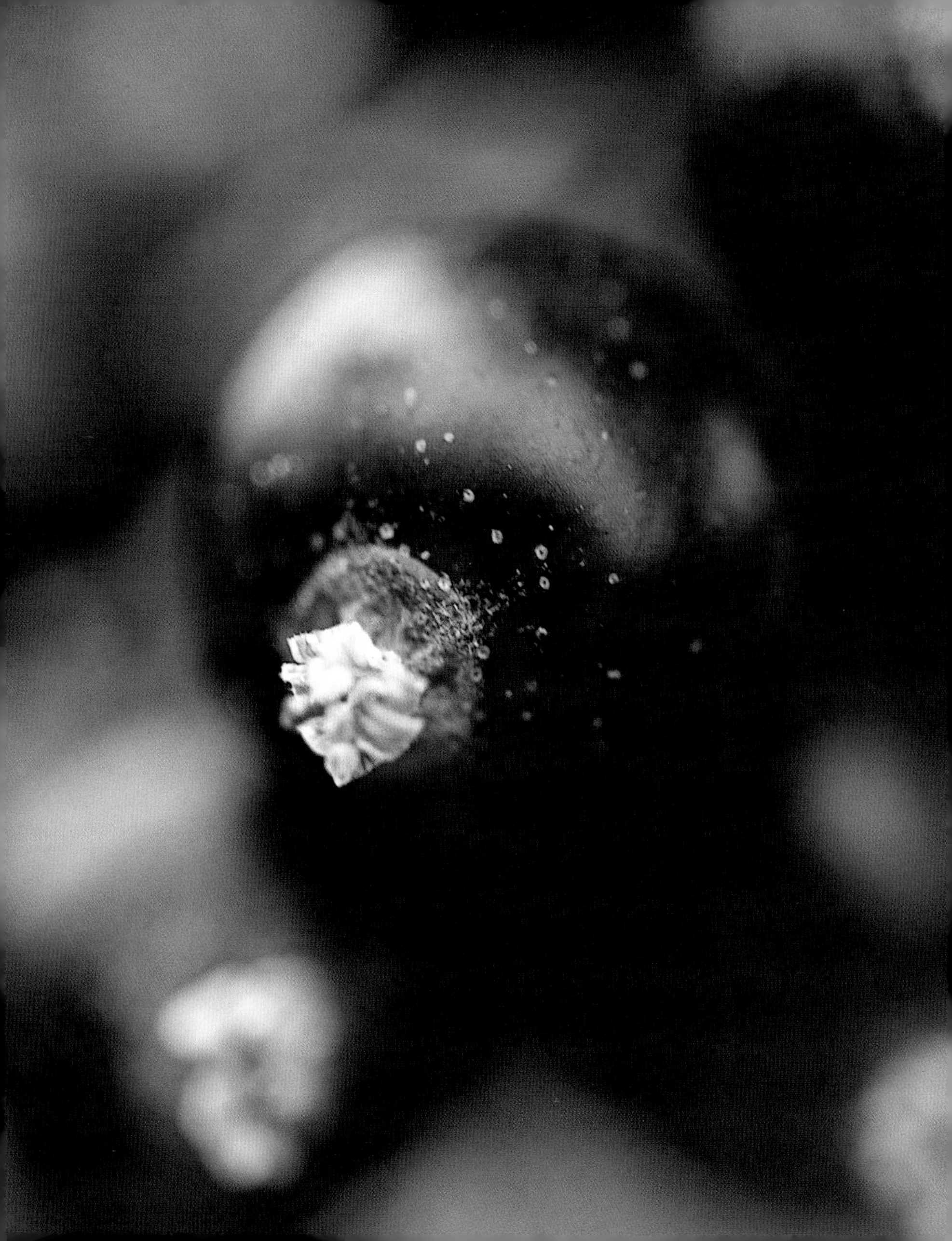

blackcurrants

Fresh blackcurrants are packed with goodness but are usually very sour, which is why popular cordial drinks are made more palatable to children with heaps of sugar. So for your little ones to benefit from the astounding immune-boosting properties of these little berries, you're best off combining them with other foods that mask the tartness. Oranges may be famous for their vitamin C content, but they only contain a third of the amount found in blackcurrants. Vitamin C is not only useful for defence against illness but also essential for healthy skin, healing cuts and grazes, responding to stress and much more. Like oranges, blackcurrants also contain vitamin C's 'companion' nutrients, bioflavonoids, which in effect prolong the usefulness of the vitamin. Bioflavonoids have a particular affinity with blood vessels – helping to keep them strong, even the tiny capillaries. The dark colour of blackcurrants hints at their rich anthocyanin content. These powerful antioxidants not only help ward off coughs and colds, but also help protect against more serious conditions such as eye problems, heart disease and cancer.

black banana pancakes

YOU DON'T HAVE TO WAIT UNTIL SHROVE TUESDAY FOR THESE – THEY MAKE A GREAT WEEKEND BREAKFAST. BUCKWHEAT CAN BE A BIT OF AN ACQUIRED TASTE, SO MAKE SURE YOU HAVE POPULAR FRUITS TO TOP THE PANCAKES WITH IF IT'S A NEW ADDITION TO THE FAMILY DIET.

FOR THE PANCAKES
100g ***buckwheat*** *flour*
pinch of salt
1 ***egg***
150ml milk or ***soya*** *milk*
100ml water
splash of olive oil, plus extra for cooking
200g ***blackcurrants***
TO SERVE
2 tbsp maple syrup
6 tbsp natural ***yoghurt***
2 ***bananas****, sliced*

To make the pancake batter, put the flour and salt into a mixing bowl and add the egg. Combine the milk and water in a jug. Beat the egg into the flour, gradually adding the liquid, plus a splash of olive oil, to make a smooth batter.

Stir the blackcurrants into the batter, squishing them slightly as you do so. Ideally, leave the batter to stand for at least 1 hour.

In the meantime, stir the maple syrup into the yoghurt and set aside.

When you're ready to cook the pancakes, lightly oil a frying pan and heat it well. Put a tablespoonful of batter into the pan and let it spread to make a thick pancake, about the size of your palm. You may be able to cook three or four in the pan at a time. Cook for 1–2 minutes until the pancakes are golden underneath, then flip over to cook the other side for a minute or so.

Serve the pancakes with a few slices of banana and a spoonful of the flavoured yoghurt.

fruit compote

YOU CAN USE ANY BERRIES, CHERRIES, APPLES, OR WHATEVER FRUIT YOU LIKE FOR THIS DESSERT REALLY.

200g ***blackcurrants***
2 ***peaches****, halved, stoned and roughly chopped*
200g ***strawberries****, halved*
100g ***raisins***
4 tbsp ***apple*** *juice*
2 tbsp honey

Put all the ingredients in a pan, slowly bring to a simmer and stir the fruits together. Turn down to the lowest possible heat and cook very gently for about 20 minutes until the fruits are soft, even a bit mushy, and the raisins have plumped up well.

Serve this compote warm or cold, with natural yoghurt, or vanilla ice cream for a treat.

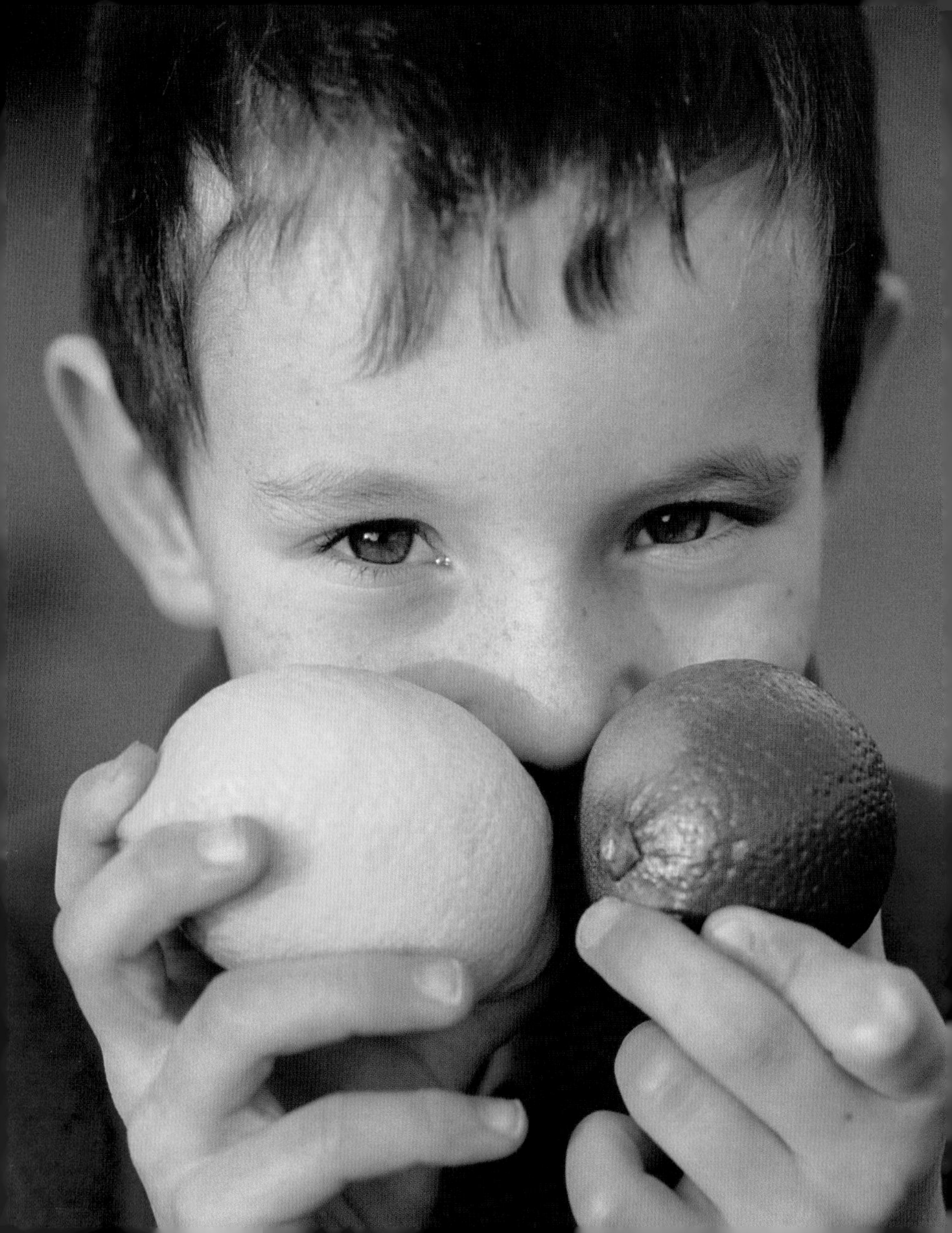

lemon & lime

Rubbing lemon or lime juice on freckles was said to shrink them... as though you'd want to! But on a factual note, it was their daily rations of this vitamin C-rich juice that helped English sailors ward off scurvy and gave them the nickname 'limeys'. Even without getting to that condition, low levels of vitamin C leave your child's health in an unfortunate state. Immune-wise, vitamin C boosts the activity of white blood cells and enhances the response of interferon (against viruses) and antibodies. It is this that makes lemon and lime juice popular for relieving coughs and colds; the citric acid is said to help purge a fever. Many lesser-known chemicals in lemons and limes, such as limonins, eriocitrin and hesperidin, are powerfully antioxidant, helping to protect children against the effects of pollution, and shown to have some anti-carcinogenic properties. Their bitterness also stimulates digestion. Contrary to what you'd expect from such acid-tasting fruits, lemons and limes are beneficially alkaline when processed in the body. Both fruits add a wonderful tangy flavour to countless dishes.

tangy tropical salsa

THIS LIVELY SAUCE GOES WELL WITH PLAINLY GRILLED FISH OR CHICKEN, OR PERHAPS BAKED TURKEY ROLLS (PAGE 152). EVEN YOUNG CHILDREN CAN HELP WITH MIXING ALL THE INGREDIENTS TOGETHER.

1 ripe ***mango***
½ ripe ***pineapple***
2 medium ***tomatoes***
1 spring ***onion****, trimmed and very finely sliced*
5mm piece fresh root ***ginger****, peeled and grated*
1 ***garlic*** *clove, peeled and crushed*
juice of 2 ***limes*** *(see note)*
1 tbsp ***sesame*** *oil*

Peel the mango and chop it over a bowl to catch any juice, tipping the fruit in and discarding the stone. Cut the skin and core from the pineapple, chop the flesh and add to the bowl. Dip the tomatoes into boiling water to loosen the skins, then peel, chop roughly and add to the other fruit.

Add the spring onion, ginger, garlic, lime juice and sesame oil and toss all the ingredients together well. (Small children can do this.)

Serve the salsa piled on top of grilled fish, chicken, turkey or meat.

NOTE If the limes are not very juicy, squeeze an extra half.

lemon roast chicken

THE GREAT THING ABOUT THIS RECIPE IS THE 'GRAVY' THAT THE CHICKEN MAKES AS IT ROASTS, ESPECIALLY IF YOU COOK IT IN A TERRACOTTA BRICK AS I DO. COOK A LARGER BIRD AND YOU'LL HAVE SOME FOR PACKED LUNCHES THE NEXT DAY.

1 ***chicken****, about 1.5kg*
4 ***garlic*** *cloves, peeled*
2 ***lemons****, halved*
2–3 tbsp tamari (or soy sauce)
8–12 dried ***shiitake mushrooms***
handful of dried ***seaweed****, such as hijiki*
freshly ground black pepper
2 tsp ***honey***
1 mugful of boiling water

Preheat the oven to 190°C/Gas 5. Wash the chicken and put it in a roasting dish (ideally one with a lid). Slice 2 garlic cloves lengthways. Poke slits into the fleshy bits of the chicken with a sharp knife and pop garlic slices into them. Squeeze the juice from the lemons all over the chicken.

Cut the spent lemon halves into three. Push half of the lemon pieces under the skin of the chicken, put a few more inside the cavity and scatter the rest in the bottom of the dish. Pour the tamari over the chicken and rub it all over the skin.

Scatter the shiitake mushrooms, seaweed and remaining garlic cloves around the chicken and grind black pepper all over it. Stir the honey into the mug of boiling water and pour into the dish.

Cover and roast in the oven, basting the chicken every 20 minutes, for 1¼–1½ hours, or until the juices run clear when you pierce between the thigh and the body with a skewer. Rest for 15 minutes.

Serve with the 'gravy', green veg and Sweet roast veg (page 45) or Squish squash (page 32).

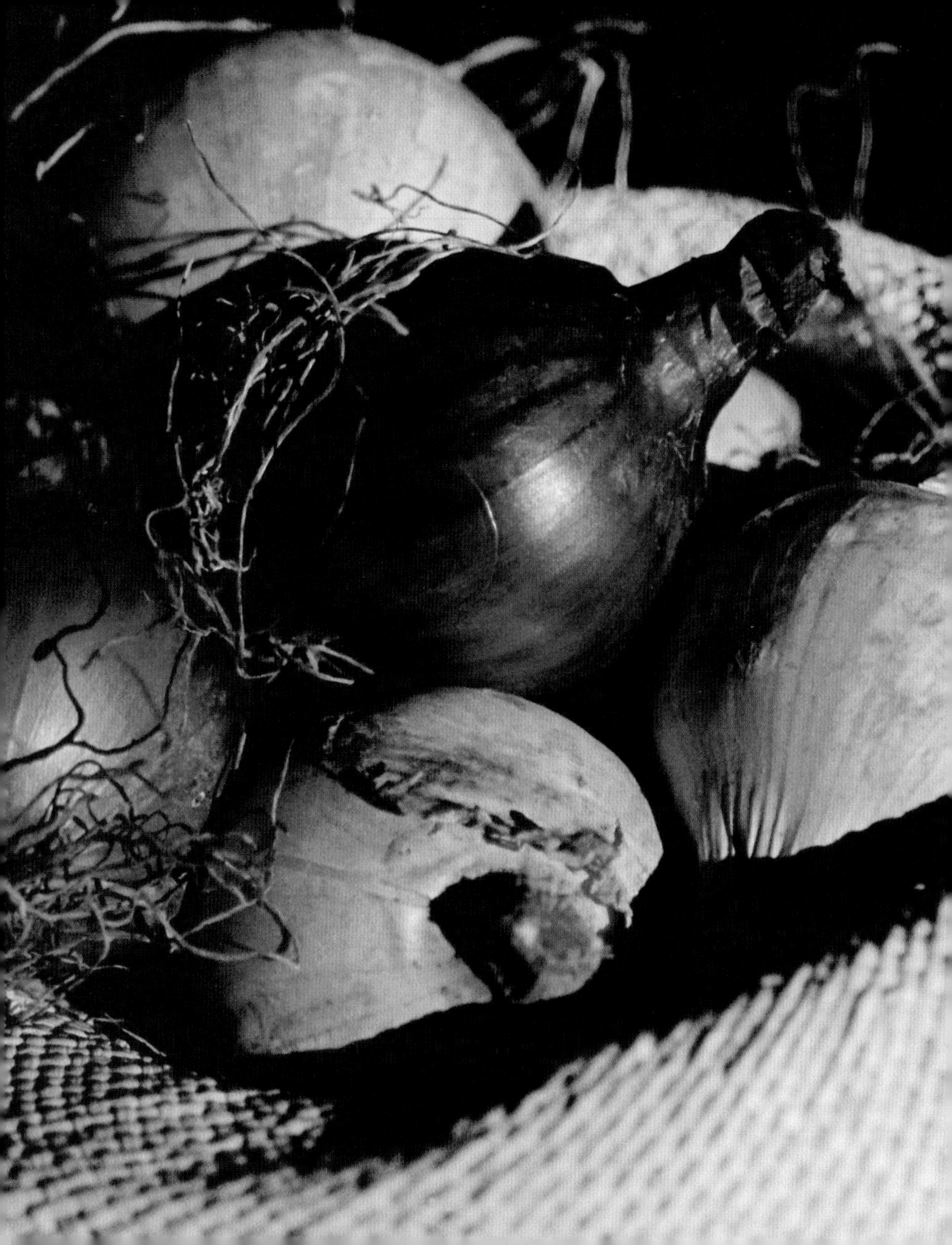

onion

Although a staple of the poor for millennia, onions were prized by ancient Egyptians as a symbol of eternal life – pharaoh Ramses IV was mummified with them in his eye sockets! Even the medicinal properties of onions have been valued for centuries. Substances such as allicin in onions have strong antibacterial action, and can help kill worms or other parasites in the intestines. Onions are also useful in helping balance blood sugar levels, partly due to the chromium they contain, but also a substance called allylpropyldisulphide. This isn't just important for diabetics, but also generally for helping prevent obesity and diabetes. Vitamin C, quercetin and isothiocyanates in onions make them powerfully anti-inflammatory, especially in conditions of the lungs such as coughs and asthma. An old-fashioned home remedy for insect bites and nettle stings was a sliced onion. Any benefit will at least in part be due to the onion's rich sulphur content. This vital mineral is needed for healthy skin and efficient detoxification in the liver, but also seems to be able to block the inflammatory histamine reaction.

cheesy onion soup

THIS IS PRETTY CLOSE TO THE REAL THING. YOU COULD LEAVE OUT THE TOAST AND JUST SPRINKLE THE CHEESE OVER THE SOUP IN THE SERVING BOWLS IF YOU PREFER.

2 tbsp olive oil
1 tbsp butter
500g ***onions****, peeled and thinly sliced*
2 ***garlic*** *cloves, peeled and crushed*
1 tsp ***honey***
1.5 litres stock (any you like, but beef stock is traditional)
1 heaped tbsp medium ***oatmeal*** *(or ground porridge* ***oats****)*

TO SERVE

4 thick slices of brown baguette
50g Gruyère cheese, grated

Heat the olive oil and butter in a large saucepan over a low heat. Add the onions with the garlic and honey and cook slowly until they are soft and transparent but not brown. Then cover and leave on the lowest possible heat for another 30 minutes until the onions are caramelised and sweet.

Pour in the stock, stir in the oats and leave to simmer, uncovered, for another 20 minutes.

When the soup is almost ready, heat the grill. Lightly toast the baguette slices on both sides, then sprinkle the cheese on top and toast until bubbling. Place a slice in the bottom of each bowl and ladle the soup over, leaving the toast to emerge as you serve!

mushroom slice

THIS SLICE IS A POPULAR VARIATION ON A POLENTA THEME – YOU CAN ADD ANY VEGETABLES YOU LIKE REALLY.

FOR THE POLENTA BASE
500ml chicken or vegetable stock
150g polenta or cornmeal
2 tbsp freshly grated Parmesan cheese
1 tsp butter
a little olive oil
FOR THE TOPPING
1 tbsp olive oil
small knob of butter
2 ***onions****, peeled and finely sliced*
2 ***garlic*** *cloves, peeled and crushed*
1 tsp ***honey***
200g ***mushrooms*** *(ideally* ***shiitake****)*
1 small courgette, cut into 5mm slices
1 tbsp chopped ***parsley***

Preheat the oven to 180°C/Gas 4. Bring the stock to the boil in a large saucepan, turn down the heat and slowly add the polenta, whisking all the time to avoid lumps. Add the Parmesan and butter as you continue to whisk. Cook the polenta, stirring regularly, until it is thick and coming away from the sides of the pan; this will take 10 minutes or so. Rub the bottom of a 23cm flan dish with olive oil, pour in the polenta and bake it in the oven for 30 minutes.

Meanwhile, prepare the topping. Heat the olive oil and butter in a large frying pan over a very low heat and soften the onions with the garlic and honey for about 10 minutes. Add the mushrooms, stir and cook for a further 20 minutes, adding the courgette and parsley for the last few minutes.

As soon as you remove the polenta from the oven, spread the mushroom mix on top of it. Cut into slices and serve immediately with a salad, such as Baby greens with raspberries (page 56).

baked veggies on toast

THIS IS A SORT OF HEALTHY, D-I-Y BRUSCHETTA! YOU COULD ADD OTHER VEGGIES, SUCH AS SLICES OF COURGETTE OR STRIPS OF RED PEPPER IF YOU LIKE, BUT THESE ONES LEND THEMSELVES WELL TO THE FUN OF BEING SQUISHED.

*2 **garlic** bulbs, broken into cloves (unpeeled)*
*12 **shallots** (unpeeled)*
*20 cherry **tomatoes***
a little olive oil
*4 slices of **rye** bread*

Preheat the oven to 200°C/Gas 6. Put the garlic cloves, shallots and cherry tomatoes in an ovenproof dish and splash with a little olive oil. Toss to coat all over, then roast in the oven for about 40 minutes.

Set the baked vegetables aside to cool slightly while you toast the rye bread.

Drizzle a little olive oil on to the toast and divide the vegetables among four plates. Get the children to squish the garlic, shallots and tomatoes out of their skins on to the toast before devouring.

veggie rice

THIS ENDS UP LOOKING LIKE A PILE OF MUSH, BUT IT TASTES DELICIOUS!

175g brown ***rice***
3 ***onions****, peeled and roughly chopped*
1 tbsp olive oil
2 ***garlic*** *cloves, peeled and crushed*
50g ***sunflower seeds***
200g frozen ***spinach****, thawed*
squeeze of ***lemon*** *juice*
freshly ground black pepper
100g feta cheese, crumbled

Cook the brown rice as directed on the packet, allowing at least 35 minutes to be sure it is tender. About 10 minutes before it will be ready, lay the chopped onions directly on top of the rice to steam. Tip the cooked rice and onions out into a bowl and keep them aside.

Heat the olive oil in the pan over a low heat. Add the garlic and sunflower seeds and stir over a medium heat for 3–4 minutes.

Add the spinach, lemon juice and pepper, then tip the rice and onions back into the pan. Stir until it is heated through and the spinach has wilted, then mix in the feta cheese. Serve immediately.

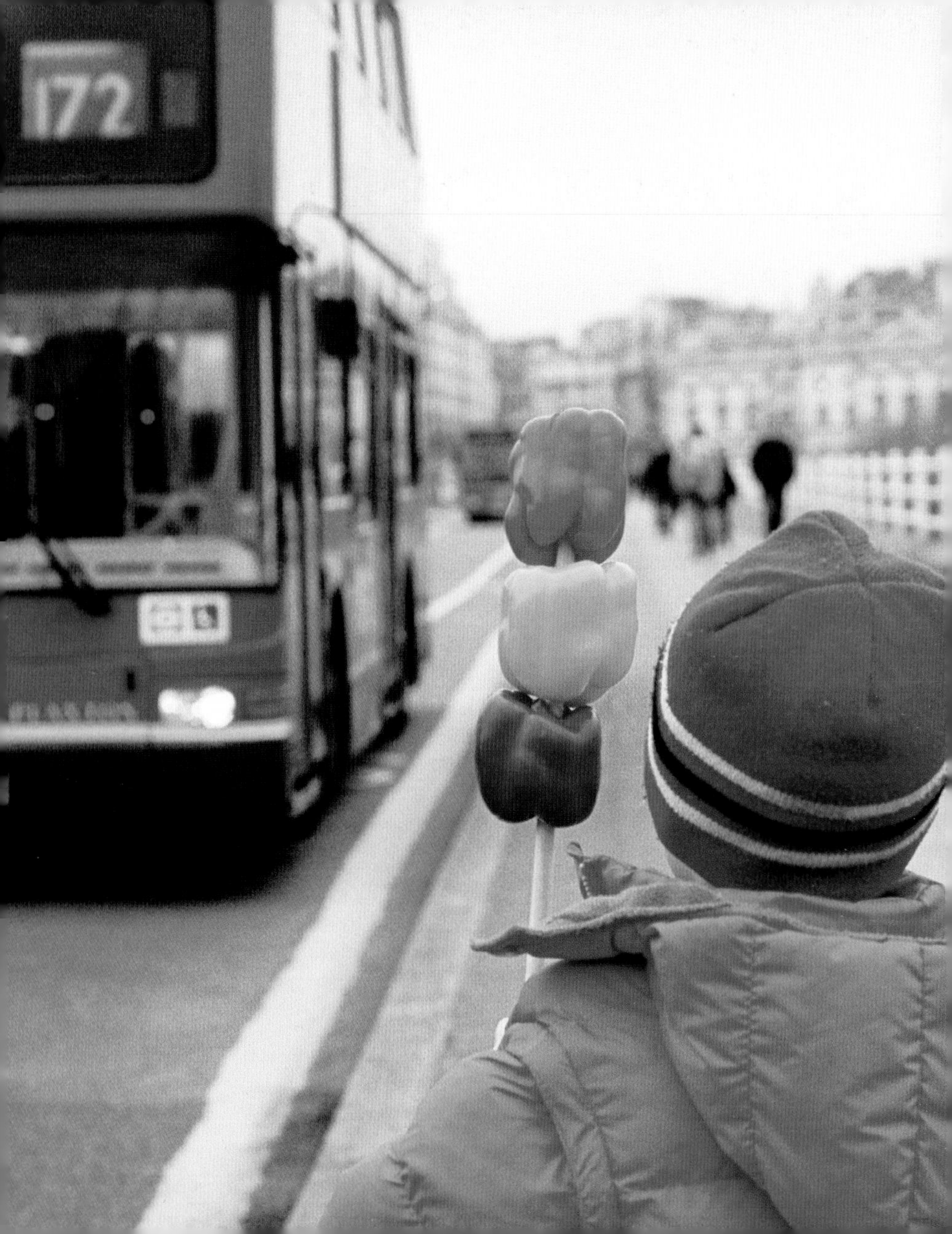
172

sweet pepper

Some children will happily eat raw peppers as finger foods from a very young age, while others need some enticing. The colouful sweetness of slow-roasted peppers will appeal to most children. All peppers are an excellent source of the immune-boosting vitamin C, as well as carotenoids such as lycopene, beta-cryptoxanthin and beta carotene (the plant form of vitamin A) that are so vital for warding off infections. Beta carotene has a particular affinity for protecting the skin, lungs and eyes. All of these antioxidants protect against the damage done within the body by free radicals from sources such as environmental pollution, cigarette smoke and eating fried foods. Peppers also contain the lesser known vitamin K, which is used for proper blood clotting and building healthy bones. Although peppers are loaded with flavour and goodness, they do belong to the nightshade family (along with potatoes, aubergines and tomatoes) and these foods can aggravate the symptoms of psoriasis, eczema, arthritis and gastric reflux in some children.

sweet pepper sauce

THIS SAUCE IS AKIN TO A SWEETER VERSION OF A BASIC TOMATO SAUCE AND CAN BE USED IN THE SAME WAY – ON PASTA OR RICE, AUGMENTED WITH FISH, PRAWNS, CHICKEN, MEAT OR OTHER VEGETABLES, OR DILUTED WITH WATER AND BLENDED TO MAKE A SOUP.

3 ***red peppers***
1 small ***onion****, quartered (unpeeled)*
1 tbsp olive oil
2 ***garlic*** *cloves, peeled and crushed*
1 tsp ground coriander
1 tsp ground ***cinnamon***
200g can chopped ***tomatoes***

Preheat the oven to 200°C/Gas 6. Lay the whole peppers and onion on a baking tray and bake for 30 minutes until soft. Put the peppers into a plastic bag and leave to 'sweat' for 5 minutes.

Meanwhile, remove the skin from the onion and roughly chop the flesh. Take out the peppers and remove their stalks, seeds and skin (you'll find it easy to do this under running cold water). Chop the peppers into small pieces.

Then, heat the olive oil in a large saucepan and soften the garlic with the coriander and cinnamon for a few seconds before adding the tomatoes, onion and peppers. Add a splash of water and leave the sauce to simmer for about 15 minutes.

NOTE For a smoother sauce, simply whiz the mixture using a hand-held stick blender before adding the chopped peppers.

colourful thai curry

YOU CAN USE PRETTY MUCH ANY VEGETABLES YOU LIKE IN THIS CURRY. IF YOUR CHILDREN DON'T LIKE CORIANDER, JUST LEAVE IT OUT. FOR A FULLY VEGETARIAN VERSION, REPLACE THE FISH SAUCE WITH TAMARI.

1 ***red pepper***
½ ***pineapple***
1 ***onion***, *peeled and finely diced*
2 ***garlic*** *cloves, peeled and crushed*
2.5cm piece fresh root ***ginger***, *peeled and grated*
2 tsp olive oil
handful of ***green beans*** *(about 15–20)*
600ml ***coconut*** *milk*
3 tbsp Thai fish sauce
1 lemongrass stalk, sliced into three
handful of frozen ***peas***
12–15 ***basil*** *leaves*
10–12 ***coriander*** *sprigs*

Halve, core and deseed the red pepper and cut into squares. Remove the skin and core from the pineapple, then cut the flesh into cubes.

In a large saucepan, soften the onion, garlic and ginger in the olive oil for 6–7 minutes.

Add the red pepper, pineapple and green beans, then stir in the coconut milk, fish sauce and lemongrass. Bring to a simmer and leave to cook gently for about 15 minutes, adding the peas for the last 5 minutes.

Remove the lemongrass and stir in the basil and coriander just before serving. Serve the curry with brown rice.

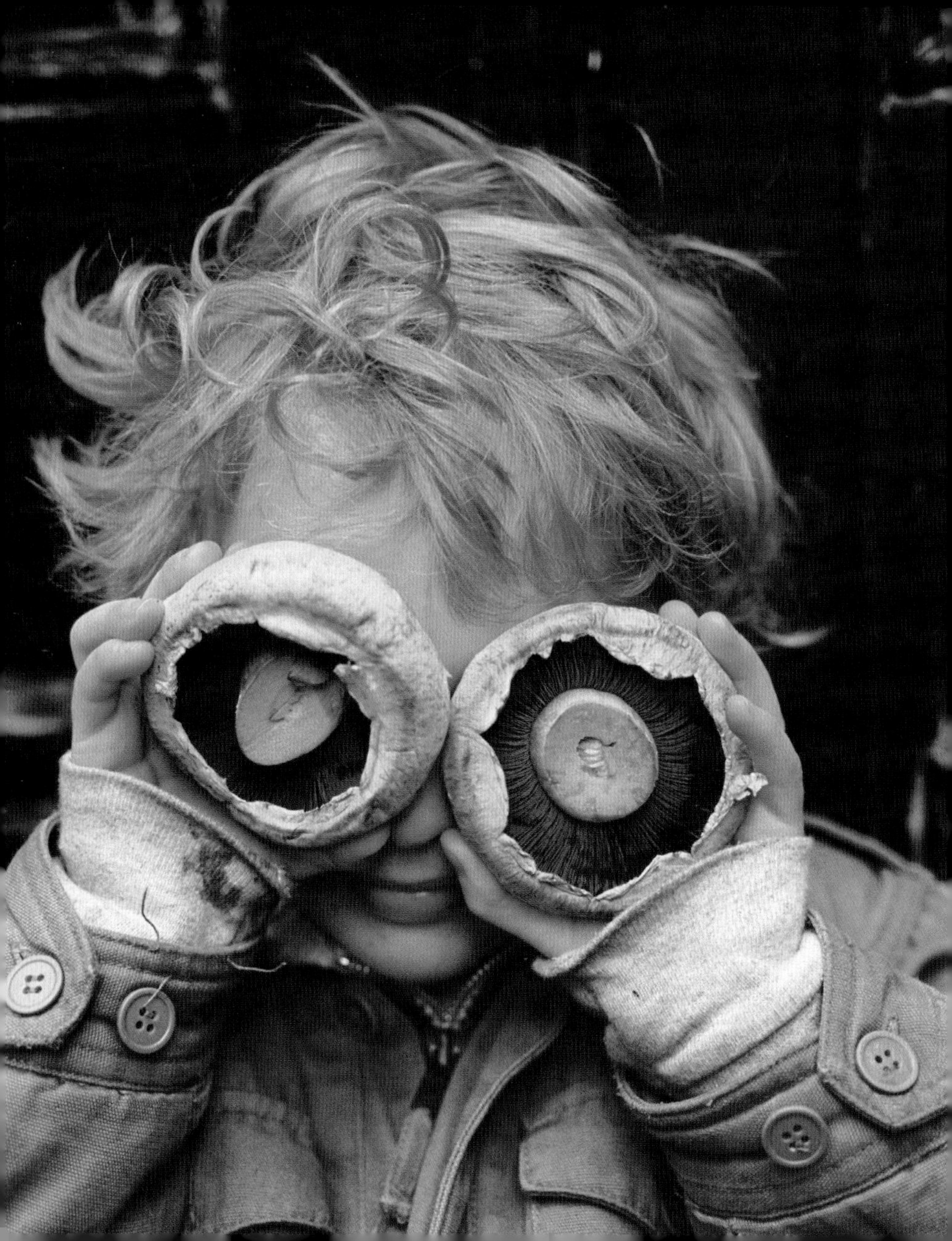

mushroom

On a recent fungal foray with a friend and her young sons, Felix and Lucian, we gathered wonderful fresh chanterelles. We were never, however, going to come across the Asian varieties such as shiitake, reishi and maitake that hog all the press for their remarkable health benefits. They have been used medicinally in Asia for millennia and research is now pointing directly to the components that stimulate immunity and help protect against heart disease. One such compound in these mushrooms is lentinan, which has been shown to enhance 'natural killer' cells and the production of the anti-viral agent, gamma interferon. In Japan it's even used alongside chemotherapy to treat cancer patients and widely used to treat people with HIV. Lentinan also, somewhat strangely given the type of plant it comes from, has antifungal properties. All this to say, these mushrooms really do pack a punch for your defences. Mushrooms also provide some protein and the vital mineral iron. If you can't buy fresh shiitake or others, get them dried – you can rehydrate them and add to risottos, soups, sauces and stir-fries.

mushroom pizzas

THE BASES FOR THESE 'PIZZAS' ARE THE GIANT MUSHROOMS THEMSELVES. USE YOUR IMAGINATION TO EXPAND THE TOPPINGS... OLIVES, ANCHOVIES, CAPERS, ARTICHOKE HEARTS, GOAT'S CHEESE AND SO ON. CHILDREN COULD SIT AROUND A TABLE MAKING UP THEIR OWN TOPPINGS.

4 large or 8 medium Portobello ***mushrooms***
4 ***shallots*** *(or 1 onion), peeled and finely diced*
1 ***garlic*** *clove, peeled and crushed*
a little olive oil
handful of leaf ***spinach****, very finely chopped*
1 tsp chopped ***parsley***
2–4 slices of Parma ham, cut in half
1–2 ***tomatoes****, sliced*
30g Parmesan cheese, freshly grated

Preheat the oven to 180°C/Gas 4. Trim the mushroom stalks if necessary. In a small frying pan, soften the shallots and garlic in a little olive oil. After 5 or 6 minutes, stir in the spinach and cook for a minute until wilted.

Lay the mushrooms, cup side up, on a baking tray and drizzle a little olive oil over the gills. Spread the cooked shallot mixture in the mushroom caps and sprinkle with a little parsley.

Trim the pieces of Parma ham so they are just smaller than the mushrooms. Layer a piece of ham on each mushroom and top with a slice of tomato.

Bake the 'pizzas' for 15 minutes. Sprinkle a little Parmesan on each one and pop them back in the oven for 3 minutes until it has melted.

khao pad gai

KHAO PAD IS JUST THE THAI TERM FOR 'FRIED RICE' THAT IS EATEN ACROSS THE WORLD – THIS IS JUST ONE VERSION, FEATURING *GAI* (CHICKEN), WHICH I ATE REGULARLY WHEN I LIVED IN BANGKOK. YOU CAN ADD PEAS OR OTHER VEGETABLES, FISH, PRAWNS OR MEAT. TO MAKE IT VEGETARIAN, LEAVE OUT THE CHICKEN, USE MORE EGG AND SUBSTITUTE TAMARI FOR THE FISH SAUCE.

200g brown ***rice***
1 boneless ***chicken*** *breast, skin removed*
1 tbsp olive oil
2 ***garlic*** *cloves, peeled and crushed*
3 spring ***onions****, trimmed and cut into 2cm slices*
1 ***red pepper****, cored, deseeded and cut into strips*
1/2 tsp smoked paprika
150g ***mushrooms*** *(ideally* ***shiitake****), quartered*
1 tbsp Thai fish sauce
1 ***egg***
sesame *oil, to drizzle*

Cook the brown rice as directed on the packet, allowing about 35 minutes, then set aside.

Cut the chicken into 1cm strips. In a wok or large frying pan, heat the olive oil. Add the chicken, garlic, spring onions, red pepper and paprika and toss over a high heat for about 5 minutes. Add the mushrooms and stir-fry for another 3 minutes.

Stir in the fish sauce, then add the rice and cook, stirring it all together for 3–4 minutes. Slowly dribble in the egg and continue to stir-fry for 2–3 minutes, or until the egg has set and the whole lot is quite dry. Drizzle a little sesame oil over the top and eat immediately.

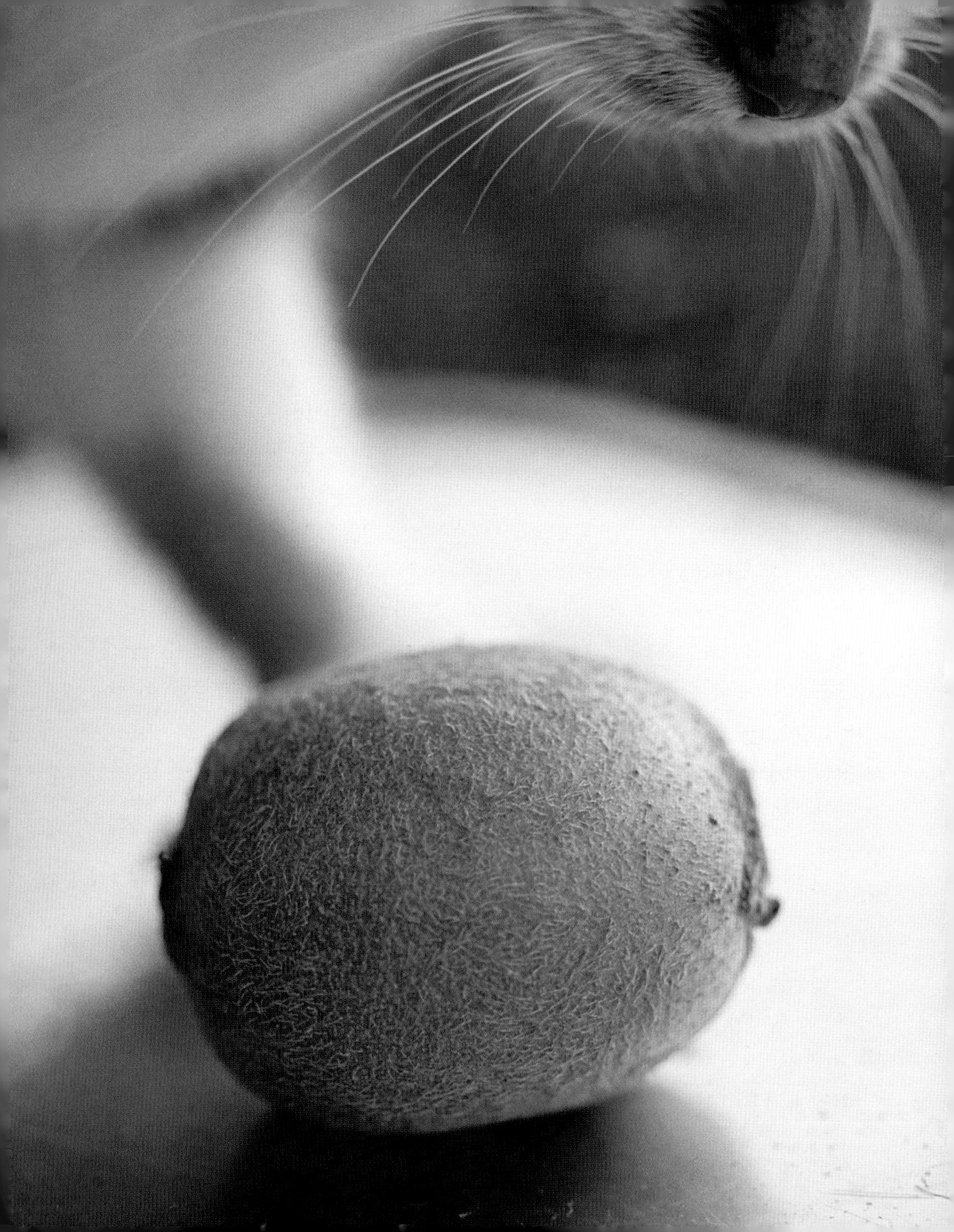

kiwi fruit

Your children may or may not like to know that the original French name for a kiwi was *souris vegetale* or vegetable mouse! Either way, the fruit's prettiness and sweet taste go down well with most children. Weight for weight, kiwis contain 50% more vitamin C than oranges and that's just one of their immune-boosting antioxidants. They also contain other antioxidant phytonutrients, including flavonoids and carotenoids, which support the body's defence mechanisms and protect against the damaging effects of free radicals. Scientists in Italy found that children who ate more kiwi and citrus fruit were less prone to wheezing and respiratory symptoms. Kiwis also contain potassium, needed to balance water, acidity, blood pressure and the function of nerves and muscles. Like most fruits, kiwis are a good source of lubricating fibre, which helps make stools easier to pass and feeds your child's beneficial gut bacteria. Also on the digestive front, they contain actinidin, an enzyme that helps break down protein. Some children, however, have allergic reactions to kiwi fruit, especially from the skin.

kiwi lollies

ONE OF THESE LOLLIES GIVES A MASSIVE HIT OF VITAMIN C AND ENERGY – AND THEY'RE NOT RESTRICTED TO CHILDREN. EVEN LITTLE ONES CAN HELP PUT THE FRUITS INTO THE BLENDER.

*4 **kiwi fruit**, peeled and sliced*
*1 **banana**, cut in half*
*2 handfuls of **strawberries**, hulled*
*juice of 2 or 3 **oranges** (about 120ml)*
TO ASSEMBLE
4 ice-lolly moulds
4 lolly sticks

Put all the fruits in a free-standing blender with the orange juice and whiz until smooth.

Pour the mixture into the moulds and freeze with lolly sticks in place for a few hours or overnight until solid before eating.

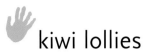

rainbow fruit salad

WONDERFOODS A-GO-GO IN THIS COLOURFUL SALAD... USE ANY FRUITS YOU HAPPEN TO HAVE IN THE FRUIT BOWL OR FRIDGE.

3 ***kiwi fruit****, peeled and chopped*
1 eating ***apple****, cored and chopped*
1/4 ***pineapple***
handful of ***strawberries****, hulled*
handful of ***blueberries***
6 dried ***apricots****, chopped small*
juice of 2 ***oranges***

Put the kiwi fruit and apple into a large bowl. Remove the skin and core from the pineapple and cut the flesh into cubes. Add to the bowl with the berries and dried apricots. Pour over the orange juice and toss all the ingredients together well.

You can serve this for breakfast, tea or dessert – it's especially good with natural yoghurt.

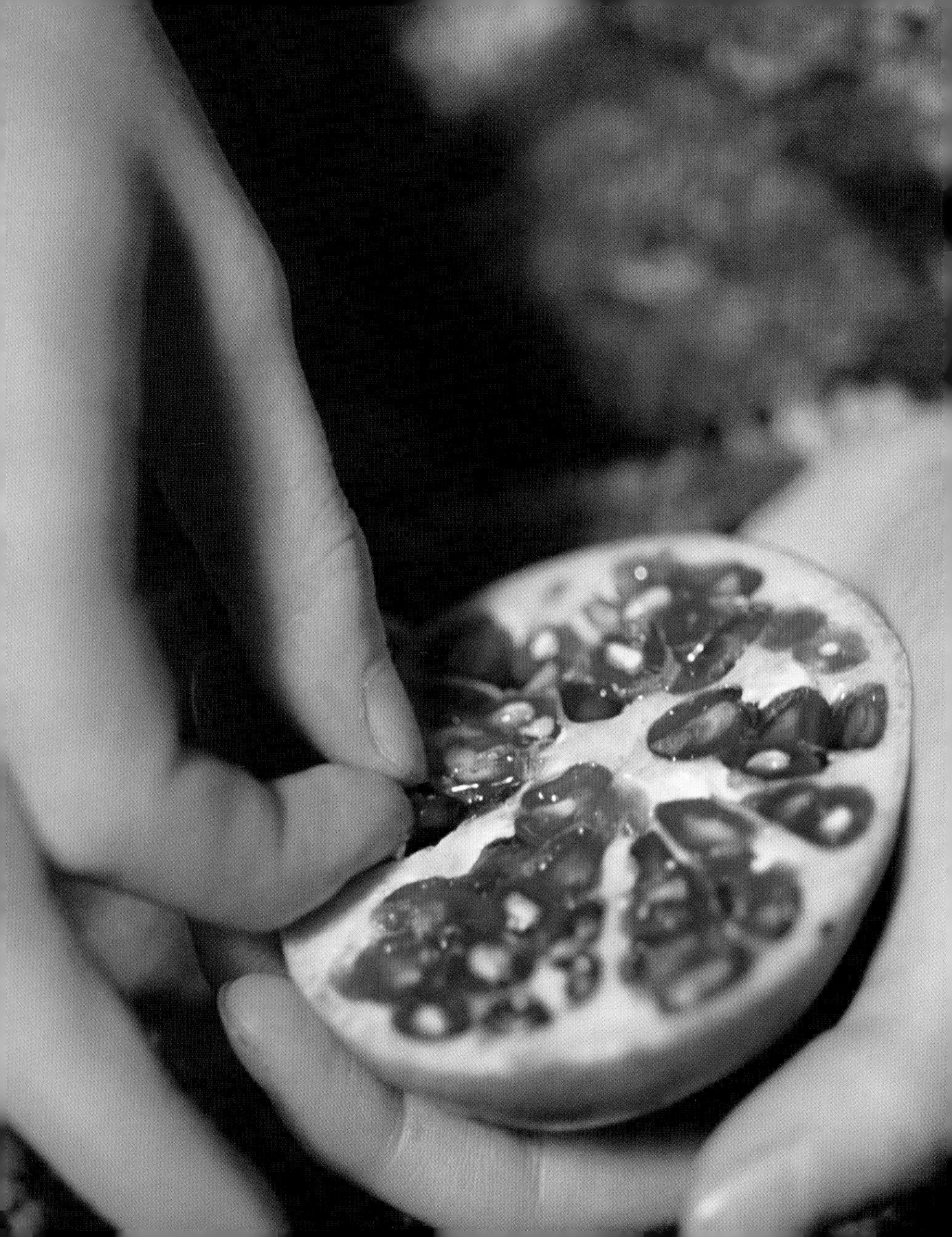

pomegranate

The word for the exploding grenade originates from the fruit, with reference to its numerous seeds that scatter as it is left to ripen. Still a luxury for most of us, the pomegranate has been valued as a symbol of abundance, fertility and life since ancient times. Traditionally, in the Middle East and India, healers used the bark, leaves and skin as well as the actual fruit to treat a wide range of illnesses from sore throats and conjunctivitis to diarrhoea. It is only in the last decade or so, though, that scientists have really investigated the fruit's amazing health properties. Pomegranates score even higher than blueberries on the broad antioxidant scale, ORAC. In particular, they are known to contain powerful polyphenols – antioxidant, anti-inflammatory substances such as punicalagin and ellagic acid, each of which acts in the body to protect against cell damage. Scientists have, however, found that it is the combined benefits of such substances in pomegranates that exert the most effect. These chemicals also protect against some of the factors that contribute to heart disease – it's never too early to start.

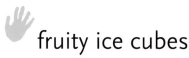

fruity ice cubes

THESE ARE A FUN WAY OF COOLING A DRINK – IN SUMMER, OF COURSE, BUT ALSO AFTER A BURST OF ACTIVITY IN WINTER, WHEN CHILDREN NEED THAT EXTRA BOOST TO THEIR IMMUNE SYSTEMS. ALTERNATIVELY, YOU COULD MAKE LOLLIES.

1 ***pomegranate****, halved*
about 350ml freshly squeezed ***orange*** *juice*
about 350ml ***apple*** *juice*
TO FREEZE
2 ice cube trays

Single out the juicy seeds from the pomegranate, putting two or three into each ice cube section. Pour over the fruit juice – orange into one tray and apple into the other. (The amount of juice suggested fits into my ice cube trays – you may need more or less.)

Put the trays in the freezer until the ice cubes are solid. Use as needed in drinks.

pick 'n' eat

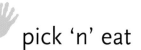

THIS IS A SATISFYING WAY TO EAT A JUICY POMEGRANATE, EASILY AVOIDING THE BITTER PITH AND MEMBRANE.

1 ***pomegranate*** *per child*
1 cocktail stick each

This is best done at a table that doesn't mind getting sticky, and in clothes that are similarly unfussy. Cut the pomegranates in half to expose the seeds.

Encourage children to eat the pomegranate seeds one at a time, using the cocktail stick to prise them out.

pomegranate & avocado salad

THIS TAKES NO TIME AT ALL TO RUSTLE UP AND YOU CAN THROW IN ANYTHING ELSE YOU FANCY, SUCH AS GRATED CARROT, SLICED CUCUMBER AND/OR SPROUTED SEEDS. JUST MAKE SURE THE AVOCADOS ARE NICE AND RIPE.

1 ***pomegranate***
2 ripe ***avocados***
about 20 seedless red ***grapes***
1 heaped tbsp ***sunflower seeds***

FOR THE DRESSING
3 tbsp olive oil
1 tbsp ***lemon*** *juice*
1 tbsp ***apple*** *juice*
1 tbsp chopped ***mint***

Open the pomegranate by making several vertical cuts through the skin and pulling the segments apart to separate out the seeds. Halve, stone and peel the avocados, then roughly chop the flesh.

Put the pomegranate seeds, avocados and grapes into a salad bowl with the sunflower seeds.

Shake the ingredients for the dressing together in a jar, drizzle over the salad and toss to mix.

Serve straight away, as a side salad with grilled chicken or meat.

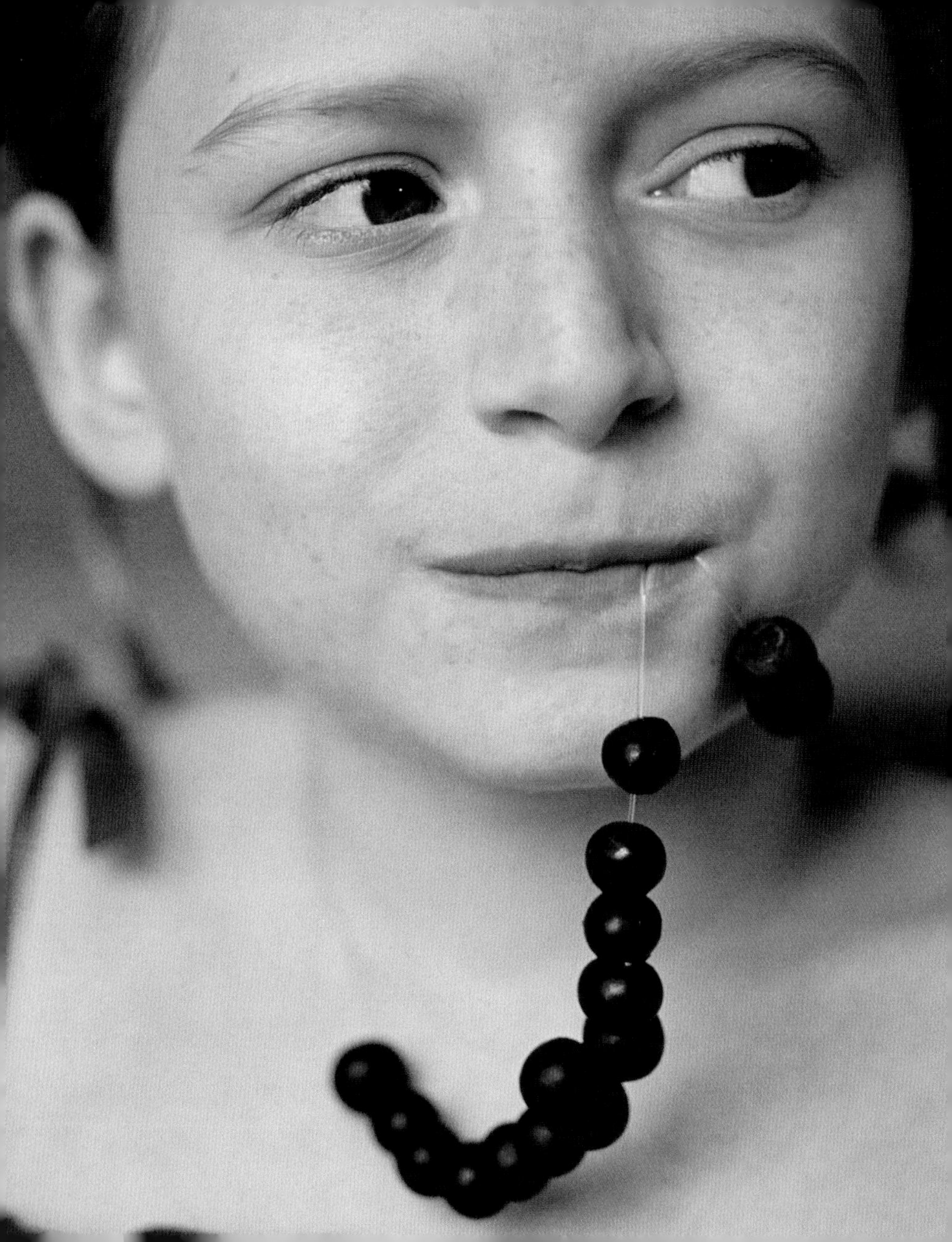

blueberries

These small, squishy berries are increasingly renowned as a wonderfood and an appealing fruit, if not a plaything for little children. For adults, blueberries are hailed as an anti-ageing miracle food, but it is those same properties that make them wonderful for children too. They are a dense concentration of antioxidants such as vitamin C and anthocyanidins, which means they offer considerable protection to the very stuff of which we are made: the ground substance in which our skin sits, all our cells and our blood vessels. Healthy blood flow means that every cell gets an efficient supply of oxygen and nutrients. The antioxidants in blueberries have a particular propensity for protecting the eyes and skin. And studies have shown that they help brain function and reduce the risk of serious conditions such as heart disease and cancer. These may seem remote considerations in children, but optimising their defences from the word go is to give them the best chance of good health. The fibre in blueberries helps to keep guts healthy; tannins can reduce inflammation and calm diarrhoea.

blue banana slush

WHO NEEDS THE ARTIFICIALLY COLOURED, OVER-SWEET STUFF YOU GET CHURNED OUT OF A MACHINE WHEN YOU CAN HAVE THIS FAR SUPERIOR SLUSH THAT IS PACKED WITH TASTE AND GOODNESS?

*200g **blueberries***
*2 ripe **bananas**, peeled and cut into chunks*
2 handfuls of ice cubes

Put the ingredients into a free-standing blender and whiz until you have a smooth, icy purée. Pour into tumblers for everyone to drink immediately.

blubbery fool

FOR SOME REASON, BLUEBERRIES HAVE BECOME KNOWN AS 'BLUBBERIES' IN OUR HOUSE. THIS IS SUCH A QUICK, CREAMY, DELICIOUS DESSERT, WHICH DOUBLES AS A FANCY BREAKFAST.

200g ***blueberries***
150ml ***apple*** *juice*
250g natural ***yoghurt***
$\frac{1}{2}$ ripe ***banana****, roughly chopped*

Put the blueberries and apple juice into a bowl and whiz to a purée, using a hand-held stick blender. Then, in another bowl, blend the yoghurt and banana together until smooth.

Put alternate layers of the blueberry purée and yoghurt in four tumblers, then using a skewer, stir it slightly to create swirls of white and purple (small children can do this).

Keep the desserts chilled in the fridge until you are ready to serve them.

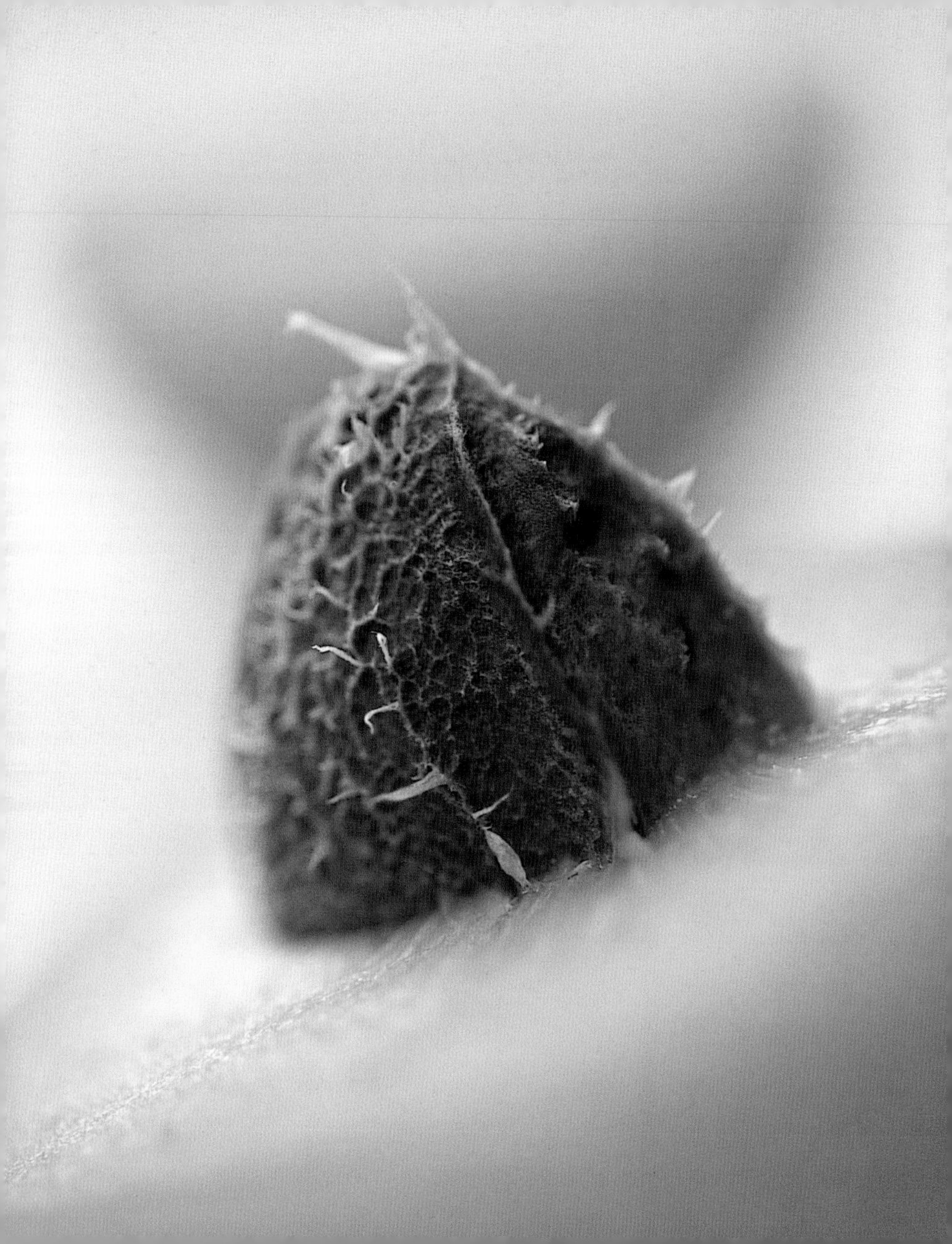

apricot

One of summer's treats – bottom-shaped, silky soft, golden with a pink blush, fresh apricots have an air of luxury about them. Their orangey colour suggests a very rich content of beta carotene, the antioxidant nutrient that is particularly important for the health of lungs, eyes and skin. So children with asthma, regular coughs, eczema and other skin problems could benefit from having apricots regularly. Talking of regular, apricots, particularly dried, are loaded with fibre – great for keeping the guts moving and ferrying wastes out of the body efficiently. Clear intestines are also useful for clear skin, as teenagers with spots will find. Dried apricots also have good levels of iron, which is important for healthy blood cells, particularly for girls who have started their periods. Both fresh and dried apricots make great snacks for children. You can also use them (and canned apricots) in desserts, smoothies and Middle Eastern-style savoury dishes. Most dried apricots are preserved with sulphur, which can trigger reactions in some children, so it's worth seeking out the darker, unsulphured ones.

sweet apricot chicken

THE SWEETNESS OF THE DRIED APRICOTS IN THIS DISH MAKES IT A FAVOURITE WITH CHILDREN. YOU COULD ADD A FEW DATES TOO, IF YOU LIKE.

½ ***onion****, peeled and sliced*
1 tsp olive oil
8 ***cardamom*** *pods*
4 ***chicken*** *thighs (or breast fillets)*
2 tbsp tamari (or soy sauce)
100ml freshly squeezed ***orange*** *juice*
100ml water
100g dried ***apricots****, roughly chopped*
50g ***almonds***

Preheat the oven to 180°C/Gas 4. In a large, shallow flameproof casserole or ovenproof frying pan, soften the onion in the olive oil with the cardamom pods.

Add the chicken and cook for a couple of minutes on each side to colour lightly, before adding the tamari, orange juice and water. Stir well and let bubble for 2 or 3 minutes. Remove from the heat and stir in the apricots and almonds.

Cover and cook in the oven for 30–40 minutes depending on the size of the chicken pieces, until they are cooked through. Check by piercing the thickest part with a knife – the juices should run clear, not at all pink.

Serve with brown rice and steamed green veg.

apricot crunch clusters

THIS MAKES ABOUT 12 LITTLE CLUSTERS – IDEAL FOR TEA OR LUNCHBOXES. YOU CAN, OF COURSE, USE OTHER DRIED FRUIT AND NUTS AND/OR ADD SOME SEEDS.

100g dried ***apricots****, cut into small pieces*
50g pecan ***nuts****, roughly broken*
150g porridge ***oats***
50g puffed ***rice***
100g unsalted butter
100g ***honey***

Line a 12-hole bun tin with paper cupcake cases. Mix the apricots, pecan nuts, oats and puffed rice together in a bowl.

Gently melt the butter with the honey in a small saucepan over a low heat. Pour on to the dry ingredients and stir until well coated.

Spoon the mixture into the paper cases and leave in a cool place until the clusters set.

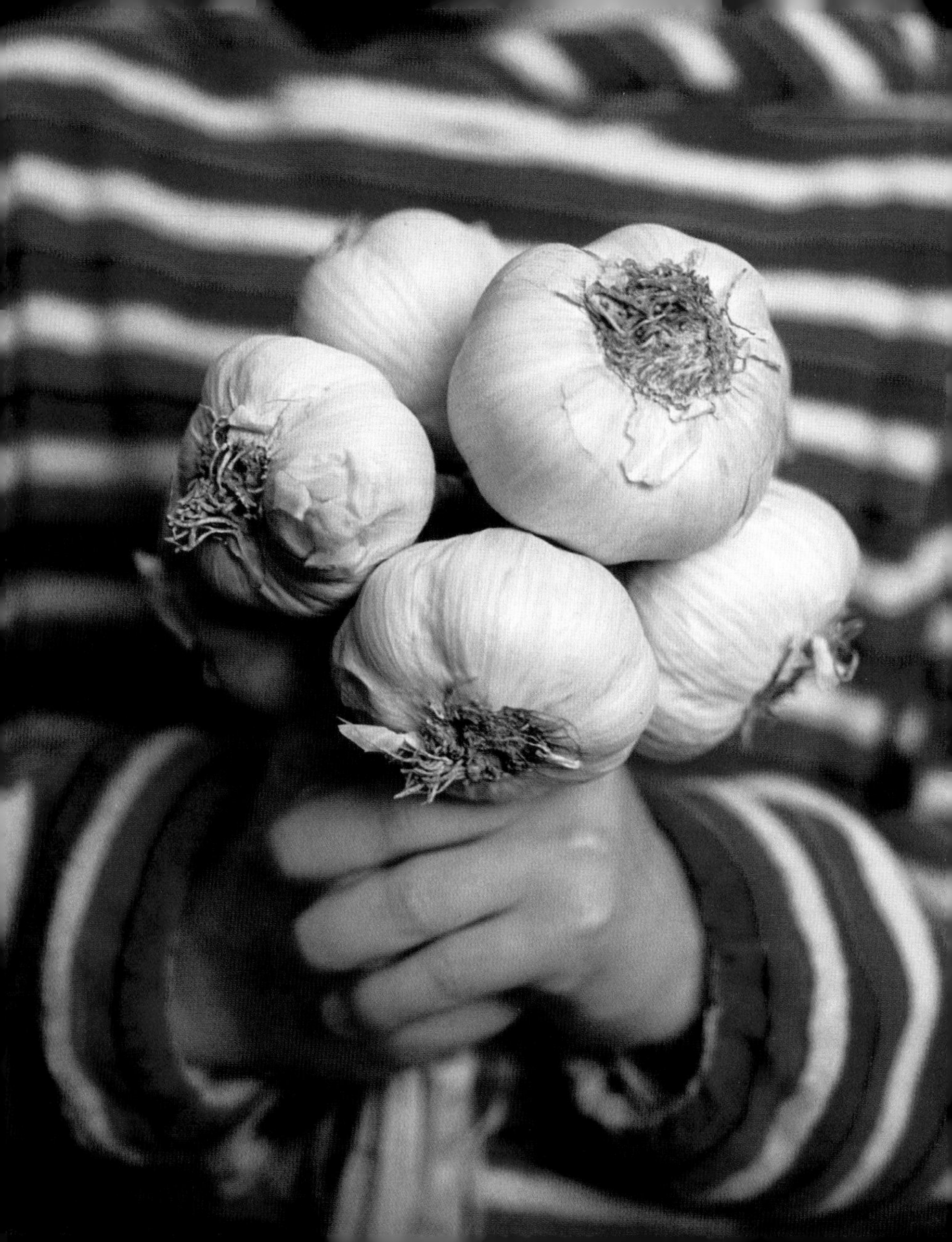

garlic

Related to lilies, garlic is nevertheless known as the 'stinking rose' and has, for thousands of years across the world, been considered something of a cure-all. It was not only esteemed for its healing properties but also for imparting strength, to the pyramid builders for example, and giving courage, not least to Roman soldiers. In terms of the body's defences, garlic is a powerful bug zapper against bacteria, viruses and fungi. It is particularly effective in the digestive and respiratory tracts with conditions such as colds, coughs, worms and tummy bugs. It is also a decongestant and expectorant, useful for stuffy noses and chestiness. All these properties are mainly due to sulphur compounds in garlic, such as allicin, which are also powerful detoxifiers for the liver and lymph system and are strongly anti-inflammatory. This last quality is particularly useful for chronic conditions such as asthma and eczema. Scientists have even found garlic to work against antibiotic-resistant strains of bacteria. Although a more remote consideration in children, the cardiovascular system benefits on many levels from garlic.

vampire pâté

IF THIS DOESN'T KEEP VAMPIRES AT BAY, NOT MUCH WILL. IT'S BEST SERVED WITH RYE OR RICE CRACKERS, PERHAPS FOR LUNCH ALONGSIDE (OR FOLLOWING) A BOWL OF POND SOUP (PAGE 22) OR ORANGEY CARROT & LENTIL SOUP (PAGE 52).

*2 cooked **chicken** breasts, boned and shredded*
4 button mushrooms, trimmed
*2 spring **onions**, trimmed and roughly chopped*
*2 **garlic** cloves, peeled and halved*
100g cottage cheese
2 tbsp olive oil
*1 tsp chopped **tarragon** (optional)*
*1 tsp chopped **parsley***
pinch of salt, to taste
freshly ground pepper, to taste

Put all the ingredients in a free-standing blender and whiz until the mixture is as smooth as you like your pâté. For a much coarser pâté, chop the chicken, mushrooms, onion and garlic very finely and mix all the ingredients together well in a bowl.

Spoon the pâté into a dish, packing it quite firmly, and chill in the fridge until ready to serve.

pad thai

ANOTHER FAVOURITE FROM MY DAYS LIVING IN BANGKOK – A NEARBY RESTAURANT NICKNAMED '*PAD THAI* CORNER' WAS ENTIRELY DEVOTED TO IT. IF YOU HAVEN'T ANY PEANUTS TO HAND (AS I HADN'T THE OTHER DAY), TOP WITH A SPOONFUL OF PEANUT BUTTER.

150g rice noodles
2 boneless ***chicken*** *breasts, skinned*
2 tbsp ***sesame*** *oil*
4 ***garlic*** *cloves, peeled and crushed*
4 spring ***onions****, trimmed and cut into 2cm slices*
8 cooked prawns, shelled and deveined
2 ***eggs****, beaten*
100g ***bean sprouts***
juice of 1 ***lime***
2 tbsp Thai fish sauce
2 tbsp sweet chilli sauce
2 tbsp roasted ***peanuts****, roughly chopped*
handful of ***coriander****, roughly chopped (optional)*

Cook the rice noodles as directed on the packet, drain and rinse them in cold water, then set aside.

Cut the chicken into thin slices. In a wok or large frying pan, heat the sesame oil, then add the chicken and toss over a medium-high heat for about 4 minutes.

Add the garlic, spring onions and prawns, then dribble in the beaten egg, stirring vigourously. Add half of the bean sprouts, closely followed by the lime juice, fish sauce and chilli sauce. Tip in the noodles and toss it all together until they are warmed through.

Divide among bowls and top with the rest of the bean sprouts, the peanuts and some coriander (if your children like it).

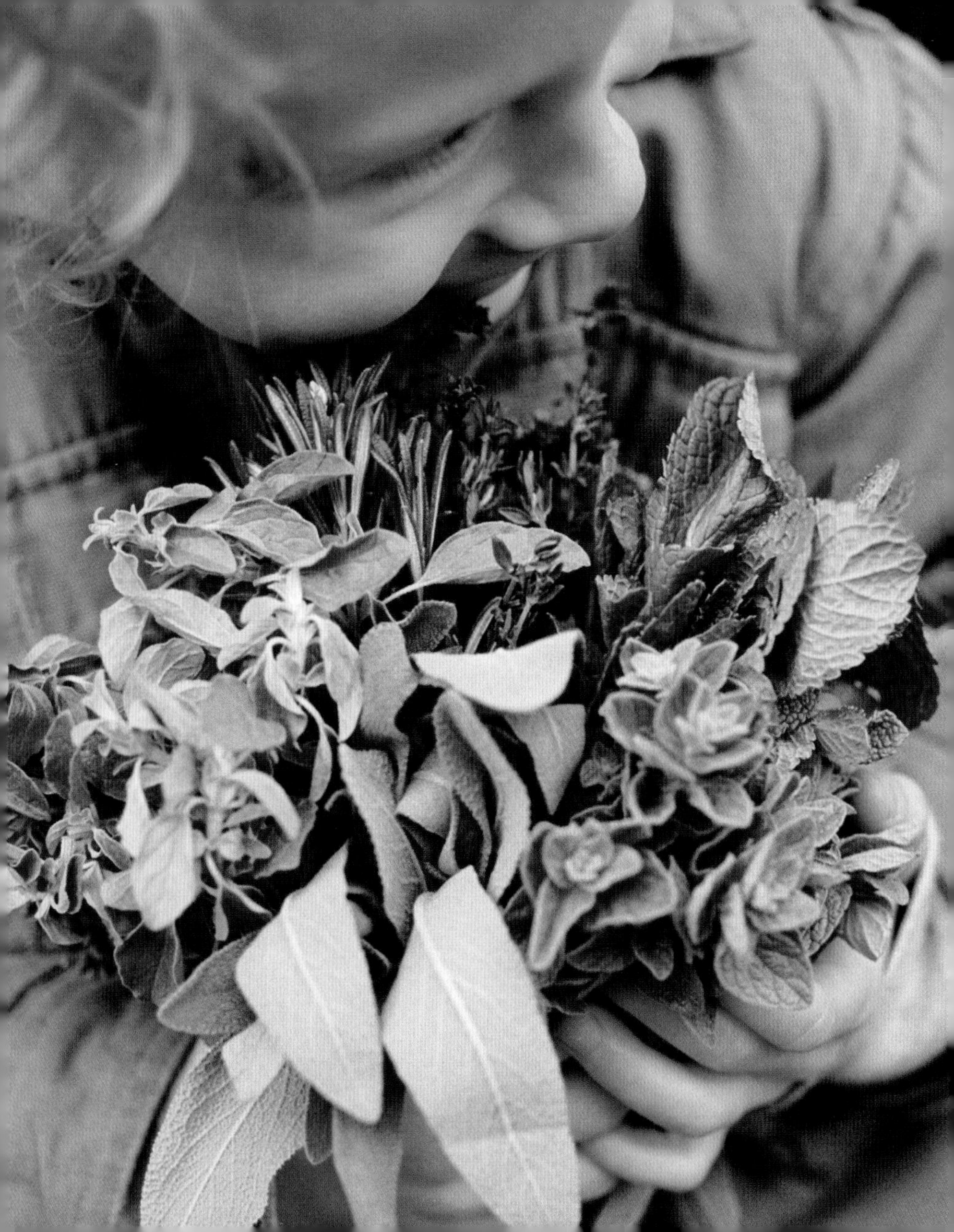

mediterranean herbs

Scarborough fair and beyond to the Med ... there is a wonderful array of herbs with which to flavour foods. Children will, of course, find some too strong or simply '*yuk*', but even a subtle scent of herbs can transform a dish and impart some health benefits. For thousands of years, herbalists have used these plants for their medicinal properties, and cooks for preserving foods. These preservation assets translate to protection in our bodies. One of the constituents in thyme, thymol, is not only antibacterial and antifungal, but also protects the fats in the brain and nerves from oxidant damage. Eugenol in basil and carvacrol in oregano, amongst other chemicals (and more in different herbs), have anti-microbial qualities that help ward off or even combat infections, including tonsillitis and tummy bugs. Rosmarinic acid in rosemary and sage are amongst many anti-inflammatory compounds in these plants. In addition to using them in freshly cooked and raw meals, a warming tea infused with sage, rosemary, mint and thyme, with perhaps a little honey, works wonders for soothing a tummy ache or cold.

turkey balls

THESE DELICIOUS LITTLE 'BURGERS' CAN BE EATEN IN A PITTA POCKET OR ON A PLATE AS A 'MEAT AND TWO VEG' MEAL. THEY GO PARTICULARLY WELL WITH THE TANGY TROPICAL SALSA (PAGE 220).

300g minced ***turkey***
2 tbsp rolled ***oats***
handful of ***parsley****, finely chopped*
5 or 6 ***mint*** *leaves, finely chopped*
1 ***tomato****, skinned, deseeded and finely chopped*
1 ***egg****, beaten*
1 tsp Dijon mustard
1 tbsp ***tomato*** *purée*

Preheat the oven to 200°C/Gas 6. Put all the ingredients into a large bowl and mix with your hands until evenly combined.

Wet your hands a little and mould the 'mush' into small rounds, about the size of a golf ball (small children can do this, just make sure they wash their hands well afterwards). This quantity should make about 12–15 balls. Lay them on a greased ovenproof tray and flatten slightly with the palm of your hand.

Bake the turkey balls for about 30 minutes until cooked through – open one up to check.

herby roast lamb

THIS GOES WONDERFULLY WITH SWEET ROAST VEG (PAGE 45) OR SQUISH SQUASH (PAGE 32). IT'S WORTH COOKING AN EXTRA LARGE LEG OF LAMB SO YOU HAVE LEFTOVERS FOR LUNCHBOXES.

1 leg of lamb, about 2kg
4 or 5 ***rosemary*** *sprigs*
generous handful of ***mint*** *leaves, roughly chopped*
3 ***garlic*** *cloves*
1 tbsp olive oil
pinch of sea salt
freshly ground black pepper
1 mugful of water
2 tbsp tamari (or soy sauce)

Preheat the oven to 190°C/Gas 5. Trim excess fat from the lamb. Strip the leaves from two of the rosemary sprigs and chop them. Using a pestle and mortar (or small food processor), mix the chopped rosemary, mint, garlic, olive oil and salt to a paste.

Lay the rest of the rosemary sprigs in a roasting dish (I use a terracotta brick with lid) and place the lamb on top. Poke slits in the meat with a sharp knife and push some of the herb-garlic mash into the holes. Rub the rest over the top of the meat and grind black pepper all over it.

Pour the mugful of water and tamari around the lamb. Roast in the oven, allowing about 45 minutes per kg and basting the meat every 20 minutes with the pan juices. When you take it out of the oven, leave the roast to rest, covered, in a warm place for 15 minutes before carving.

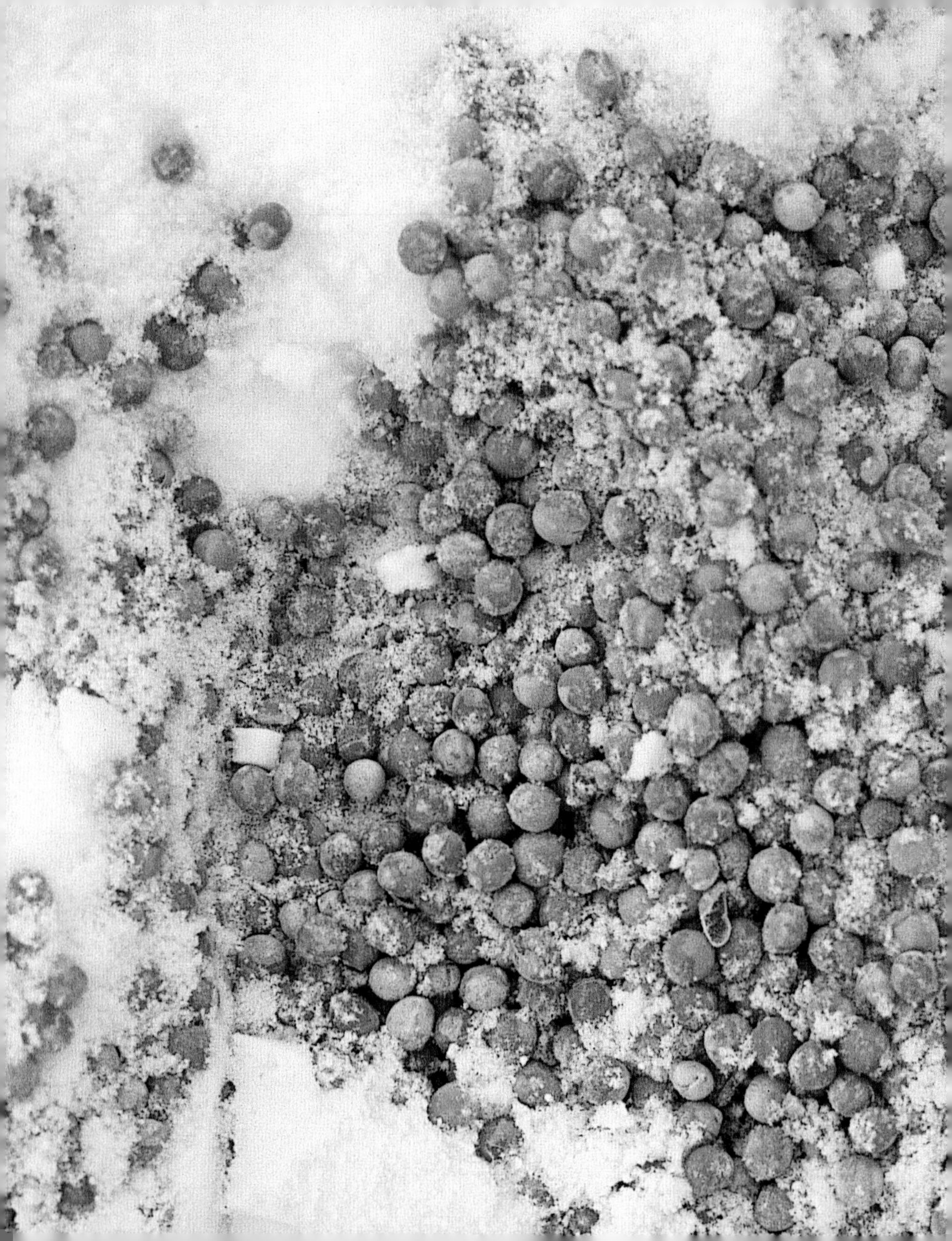

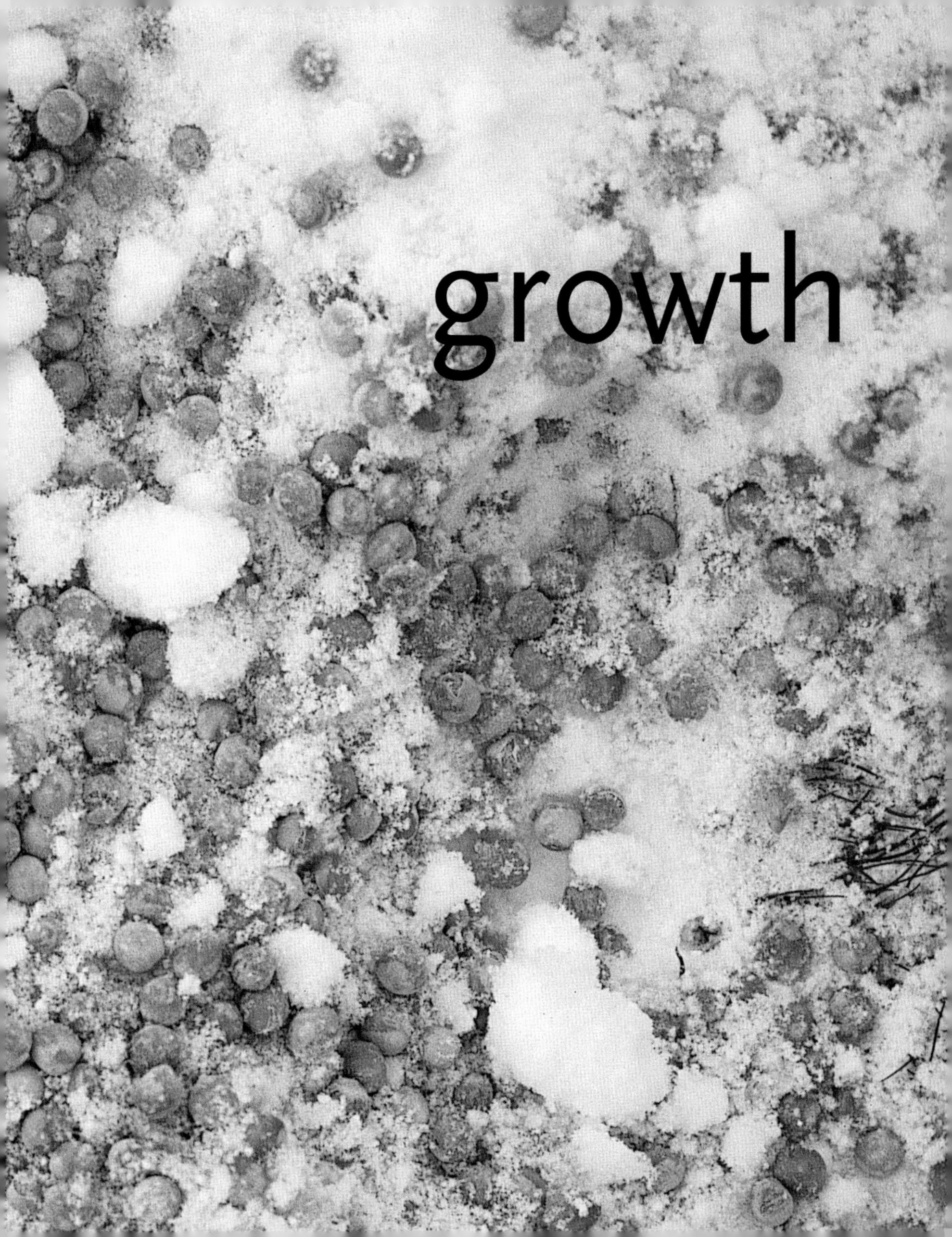

growth

Almost as much as I dreaded her 'friendly' pinch of my cheek each time I saw her, the predictability of my Great Auntie Margot's "Haven't you grown!" exclamations was a groan-worthy ritual. It can't help but be one of the first things you notice about a child you haven't seen in a while, but for many children such remarks on changes in their bodies becomes an embarrassing bore. Yet for others, who are in a fallow growth period, they just long to hear such words. The fact is though, that children grow in fits and starts and a slow growth period is rarely much to worry about.

In order for children to grow and develop appropriately, they need a whole range of nutrients, not to mention other less tangible things like exercise, mental stimulation and loving care. The wonderfoods throughout this book and particularly in this chapter contain the full range of nutrients they need: macronutrients, i.e. the ones they need in larger amounts – protein, carbohydrates and fat. They also need the full spectrum of micronutrients, i.e. vitamins, minerals and other substances that are essential, not just for the production of new cells for growth, but also for all of a child's mental faculties to develop and for all-round good health.

Scientific research has shown that children brought up on a vegan diet are at risk of not growing properly if that diet is poor and sufficient care isn't taken to ensure they get the full range of nutrients. A vegan diet is inherently deficient in the crucial vitamin B_{12} so if you are raising your child on an animal-free diet, it's worth getting well informed and talking to a health professional about supplementation. It's also important to make sure that he or she gets enough quality protein and is able to digest plant-source proteins well. With vegetarian children, it is easy to fall back on cheese as a regular protein, at the expense of beans and lentils, which feature in other sections of this book. Given a broad, healthy diet, there is no reason why a vegetarian child cannot develop as well as any other and may even have a lower risk of certain diseases.

A vital nutrient for growth is zinc, which is found not just in fish but also in pumpkin seeds as well as other wonderfoods throughout the book. Folic acid is best known for helping to prevent spinal tube defects in unborn babies, but it is needed throughout life for cell replication and growth. It helps make the building blocks of DNA, the body's genetic blueprint. Several of the foods in this chapter contain folic acid.

The wonderfoods in this chapter will not, alone, make your child grow. Rather, as part of a varied diet, based on all the wonderfoods, they have some particular nutrients that are vital for proper development.

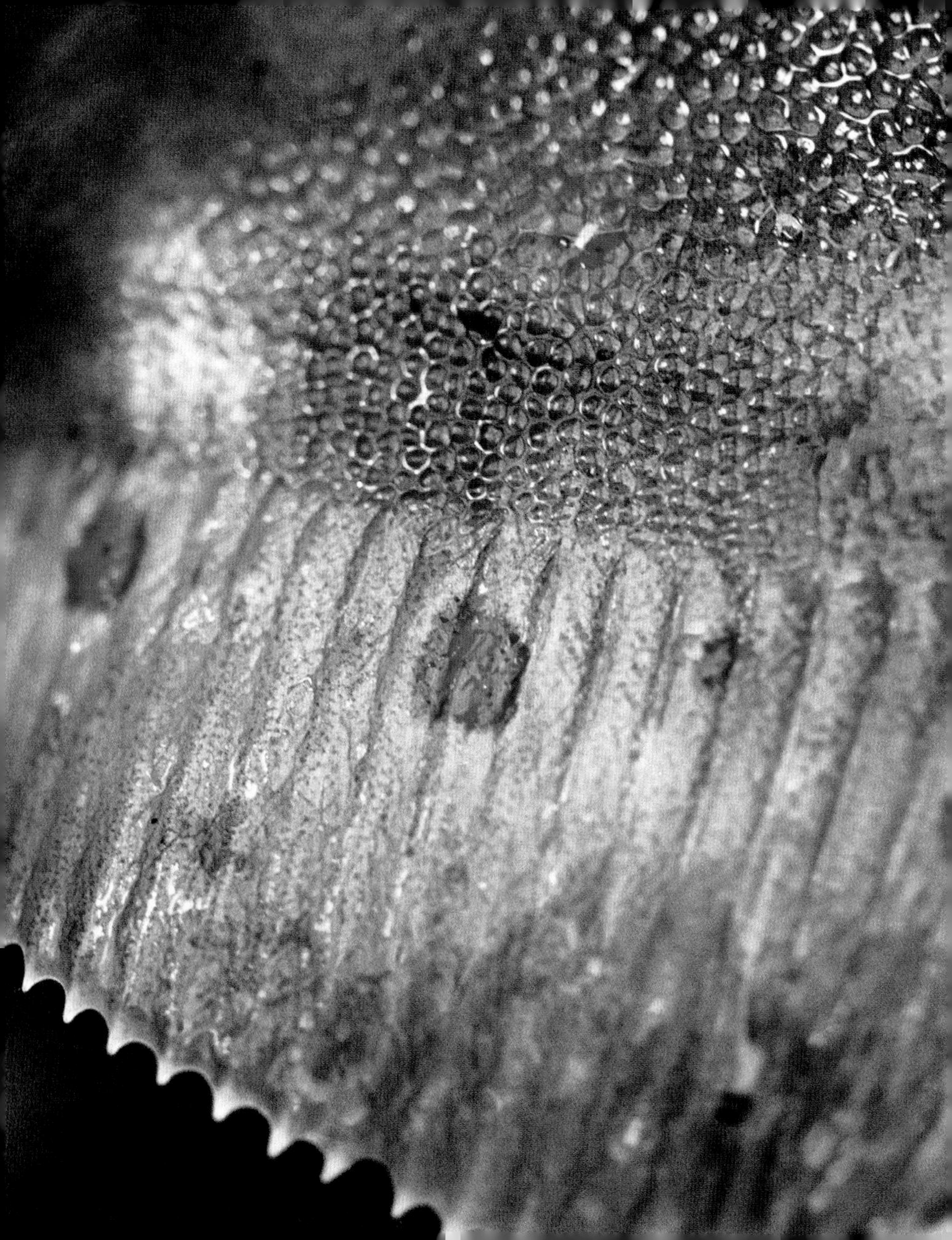

white fish

Fish is about as perfect a protein as you can give your children. Not only does it provide all the amino acids needed for building a healthy body, but it is relatively easily digested and any fats it contains are beneficial ones. Government recommendations are for at least two portions each week, yet a shocking seven out of ten people in the UK don't even have fish once a week. Children need a regular intake of healthy protein to fuel their ongoing growth and development. It also means that a meal is more sustaining in terms of energy release. In addition to protein, fish contains good levels of B vitamins, particularly B_3, B_6 and B_{12}, which are all needed for proper cell replication (for growth and repair), energy production and balanced moods, amongst countless other things. The mineral, selenium, in fish is an important antioxidant that helps block the uptake of toxic substances such as lead and mercury from the environment, to which your child may be exposed. And even white fish like cod contain some omega 3 fats, which are useful for combating the inflammation of asthma and eczema.

mini fish & chips

HERE'S THAT TRADITIONAL BRITISH FAVOURITE WITH A FEW TWISTS AND NOT A DEEP-FRYER IN SIGHT.

500g potatoes (any you like)
olive oil, for cooking
500g haddock, cod or other chunky, ***white fish*** *fillet*
2–3 tbsp cornflour
1 tbsp ***sesame seeds***
1 ***egg****, beaten*

Preheat the oven to 190°C/Gas 5. Cut the potatoes into wedges (no need to peel) and put them on a baking tray. Splash with a little olive oil, shake to coat all over and put into the oven. Bake for about 40 minutes, depending on the size of the wedges, until they are crisp, golden and cooked through.

Meanwhile, check the fish is free of small bones, then cut into bite-sized pieces. Now coat the fish for frying (small children could do this). Put the cornflour and sesame seeds in a bowl and toss to mix. One by one, dip each piece of fish in the beaten egg, then quickly roll in the flour mix to dust all over.

When the potatoes are almost done, heat 2 tbsp olive oil in a wok or large frying pan. Add a handful of coated fish pieces (just enough to cover the bottom of the pan) and cook for 4–5 minutes, turning them regularly. Drain on kitchen paper while you cook the rest in the same way. Serve the fish and chips with peas.

fish pie with sweet mash topping

A TASTY COMBINATION OF SEAFOOD IN A CREAMY LEEK SAUCE UNDER AN INVITING SWEET POTATO AND SWEDE MASH TOPPING. REMEMBER TO CHECK THE FISH FOR ANY SMALL BONES BEFORE YOU CUT IT UP.

*400g **sweet potatoes** (about 3 medium), peeled*
300g swede, peeled
knob of butter
*450ml milk or **soya** milk*
1 tbsp olive oil
1 medium leek, washed and thinly sliced
2 tsp cornflour (see note)
1 tsp Dijon mustard
sea salt and freshly ground black pepper
*1 small head of **broccoli**, cut into small florets*
*200g filleted **salmon** or chunky **white fish**, cubed*
*100g undyed smoked **haddock**, cubed*
100g prawns, shelled and deveined

Preheat the oven to 180°C/Gas 4. Cut the sweet potatoes and swede roughly into cubes and put into a large saucepan. Add water to cover and boil for about 10 minutes until soft enough to mash. Drain well and tip into a bowl. Add the butter and about a quarter of the milk and mash well (young children can do this). Set aside.

In another pan, heat the olive oil and cook the leek for 4–5 minutes. Stir in the cornflour and slowly dribble in the rest of the milk, stirring continuously. Add the mustard and seasoning, followed by the broccoli, fish and prawns. Stir it altogether well for a couple of minutes.

Tip the mixture into a baking dish (I use a deep 23cm round dish) and cover it evenly with the mash. Bake in the oven for 25 minutes.

NOTE If you haven't any cornflour in the kitchen, use 2 tbsp of ground-up oats instead.

fish teriyaki

HUNT OUT MIRIN AT A LARGE SUPERMARKET, HEALTH FOOD SHOP OR ASIAN GROCER. THIS SWEET, JAPANESE ALCOHOL (SOMETIMES ERRONEOUSLY CALLED RICE WINE) IS A GREAT ADDITION TO MARINADES. I FIND THIS PARTICULAR MARINADE WORKS WELL WITH OILY FISH AND CHICKEN TOO.

4 ***fish*** *fillets, such as plaice or cod*

FOR THE MARINADE

2 tbsp tamari (or soy sauce)
2 tbsp mirin
3 tbsp freshly squeezed ***orange*** *juice*
1 tbsp ***sesame*** *oil*
2 tsp runny ***honey***

In a large bowl, mix the marinade ingredients together, stirring well until the honey dissolves. Add the fish fillets and slosh them around in the mixture to coat well (young children can do this). Leave to marinate for up to 20 minutes if you have enough time.

Heat a griddle pan over a high heat. Add the fish, skin side down, with the marinade, making sure the fillets lay flat. Cook without moving for 3–4 minutes, then turn the fish fillets over and cook them for about 2 minutes on the other side.

Remove the fish to warm plates, leaving the sauce to get stickier in the pan for another minute or two. Drizzle the sticky sauce over the fish and serve with brown rice. Sesame beans (page 137) also go well with this dish.

monkfish kebabs

FOOD ON A SKEWER SOMEHOW IS MORE APPEALING, ESPECIALLY TO CHILDREN, ALTHOUGH THIS WORKS PERFECTLY WELL GRILLED WITHOUT STICKS. YOU CAN ADD OTHER FLAVOURINGS TO THE MARINADE, SUCH AS SESAME OIL, OR WHATEVER TAKES YOUR FANCY. EVEN YOUNG CHILDREN CAN HELP THREAD THE SKEWERS.

400g ***monkfish*** *fillet*
1 ***red pepper***
1 ***yellow pepper***
2 courgettes, sliced into discs
4 bamboo skewers
few capers (optional)

FOR THE MARINADE

3 tbsp olive oil
juice of 1 ***lemon***
1 large ***garlic*** *clove, peeled and crushed*
freshly ground black pepper
pinch of salt

Cut the monkfish into 2–3cm cubes. In a large dish, mix all the marinade ingredients together, then add the fish cubes and toss to coat well. Set aside to marinate for about 20 minutes.

In the meantime, preheat the grill to medium. Halve, core and deseed the peppers and cut into 2cm squares; cut the courgettes into 1cm thick slices. Lay the peppers and courgettes on the grill rack, brush with a little of the fish marinade and pop under the grill for about 10 minutes to cook through a little (otherwise they will stay a bit raw on the skewers).

When the vegetables are cool enough to handle, thread them and the fish cubes on to bamboo skewers, alternating the colours. Grill the kebabs for about 3–4 minutes each side until the fish is cooked, turning and basting them with the remainder of the marinade halfway through grilling.

Serve topped with a few capers if you like, and accompanied by Spiced quinoa (on page 167) and a Wondergreen salad (page 285).

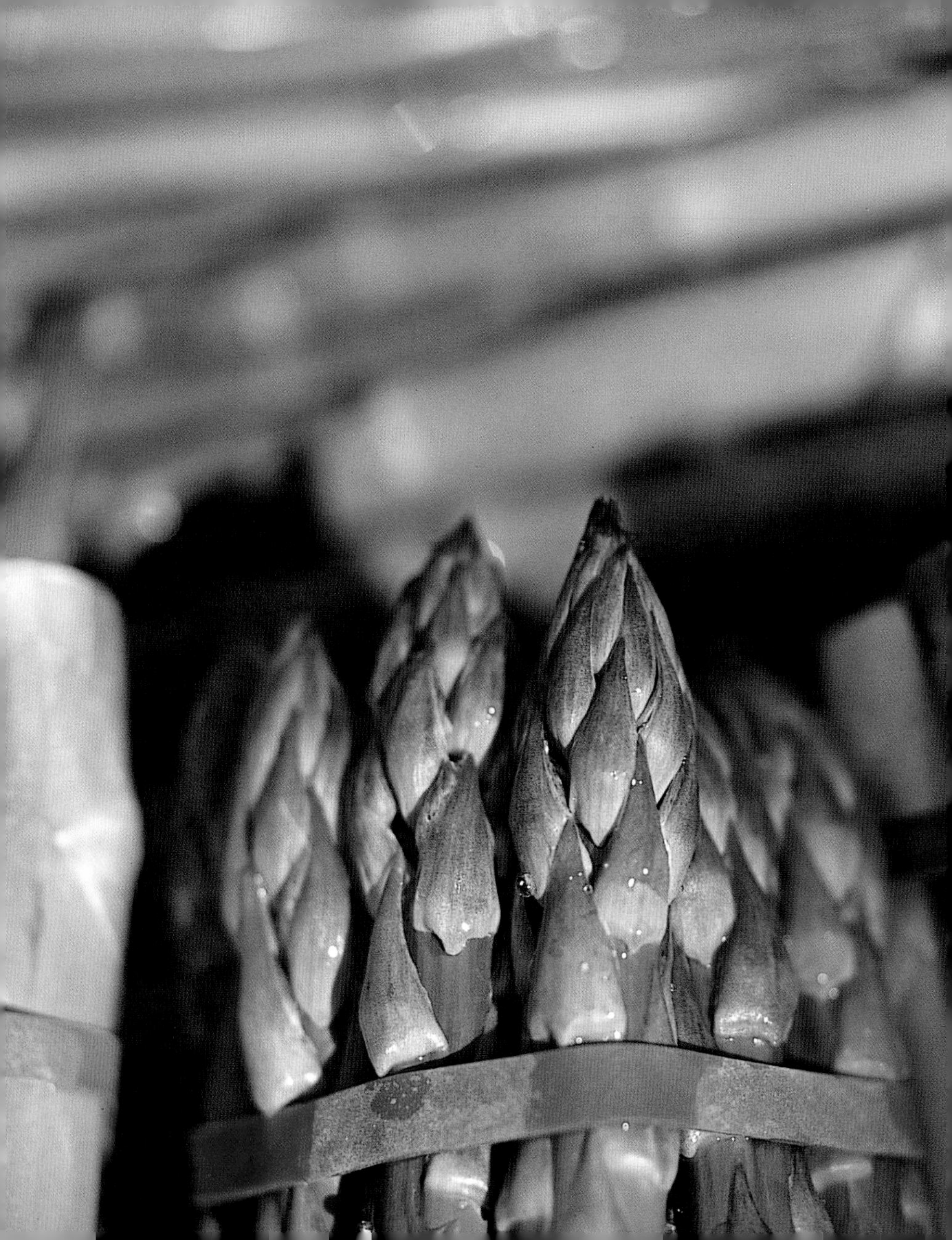

asparagus

Asparagus may be considered quite a delicacy and therefore not something usually given to children, but what was once known as 'sparrowgrass' in 18th century London, is a fun treat for children too... not least because they can eat it with their hands with impunity. Asparagus is one of the richest food sources of folic acid. This vital member of the B vitamin family is essential for the body to make DNA (our cellular blueprint) and therefore for proper cell replication needed for growth and repair. Folic acid is also needed for good cardiovascular and mental health. A hundred grams of asparagus can provide almost all of a ten-year-old child's folic acid needs for a day. An amino acid called asparagine (responsible for the strong odour in the urine after asparagus is eaten), alongside the mineral potassium, makes asparagus good for flushing wastes through the kidneys. Asparagus also contains a type of fibre called inulin, which can be used as fuel by the beneficial bacteria in the intestines. Providing these bacteria with inulin helps them to proliferate and keep your child's guts in a good condition.

spears 'n' sauce

THIS MAKES A LIGHT SUPPER IN ITSELF. YOU COULD VARY THE OIL, PERHAPS USING WALNUT RATHER THAN SESAME, AND REPLACE THE SESAME SEEDS WITH FRESHLY CRUSHED WALNUTS IF YOU LIKE.

24–32 ***asparagus*** *spears*
FOR THE DIPPING SAUCE
200g Greek-style natural ***yoghurt***
2 tbsp ***sesame*** *oil*
small bunch of chives, finely chopped
2 tbsp ***sesame seeds***

Put a large saucepan of water on to boil. Snap off and discard the woody ends of the asparagus spears; they'll find their own breaking point about 3cm from the base. (Small children can do this.)

Add the asparagus to the boiling water, tips uppermost (so they cook in the steam rather than the water), and blanch for about 3 minutes until just tender. Drain and briefly rinse under running cold water, then drain the spears well.

Mix the dipping sauce ingredients together in a bowl. Divide the asparagus spears among plates and sprinkle with the sesame seeds. Serve them with the dipping sauce.

salmon & asparagus slice

THIS IS A SORT OF QUICHE WITH A BASE OF POLENTA RATHER THAN PASTRY. IT IS BEST HOT, BUT CAN BE EATEN COLD – EVEN PACKED INTO LUNCHBOXES.

FOR THE POLENTA BASE
500ml vegetable or chicken stock
150g polenta or cornmeal
2 tbsp Parmesan cheese, freshly grated
walnut-sized knob of butter
a little olive oil
FOR THE TOPPING
6–8 ***asparagus*** *spears, trimmed*
olive oil, to drizzle
200g ***salmon*** *fillet*
3 ***eggs***
250ml milk
freshly ground black pepper
pinch of fine sea salt
½ tsp mustard powder
3 spring ***onions****, trimmed and finely sliced*

Preheat the oven to 180°C/Gas 4. Bring the stock to the boil in a large saucepan. Lower the heat and slowly add the polenta, whisking constantly to avoid lumps. Add the Parmesan and butter as you continue to whisk. Cook the polenta, stirring regularly, until it is very thick and comes away from the sides of the pan easily, about 10 minutes.

Smear the bottom of a 23cm flan dish with olive oil, pour in the polenta and bake it in the oven for 30 minutes, while you prepare the filling.

Lay the asparagus on a baking tray, drizzle with olive oil and roll to coat. Place the salmon on the same tray and bake in the oven for 10 minutes.

Meanwhile, beat the eggs, milk, seasoning and mustard together in a bowl, then add the spring onions. Flake the salmon (checking for any small bones) and cut the asparagus spears in half.

Scatter the salmon flakes over the baked polenta and lay the asparagus evenly over the top. Carefully pour over the egg mixture and bake in the oven for about 30 minutes until the filling is set. Serve with a Wondergreen salad (page 285).

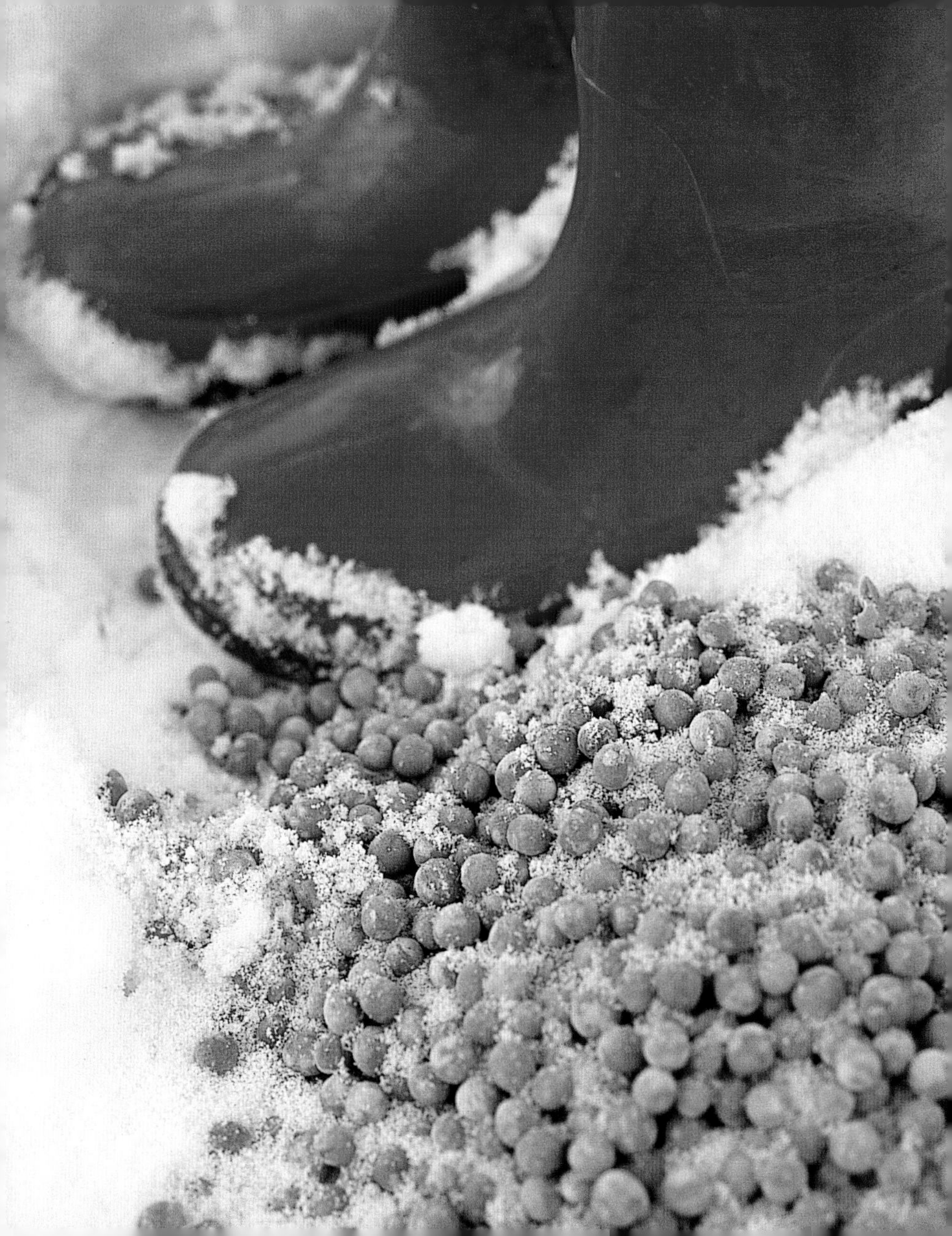

peas

Peas are just about every child's favourite vegetable, especially good when picked up squished into a forkful of mashed potato. And the extra good news – for you, if not necessarily for your children – is that they're bursting with vitamins and minerals. Peas are an excellent source of folic acid and zinc, both needed for growth in children, and of vitamin K, essential for strong bones. In addition to folic acid, peas contain a range of other vitamins from the B family – B_1, B_2, B_3 and B_6 – all needed for growth, energy production, repair, digestion and hormone balance. Peas also provide very good levels of protein, fibre and vitamin C. Their beta carotene, along with the zinc and vitamin C, contributes to a child's immunity, helping keep infections at bay. They also provide iron, which is so essential for healthy red blood cells – a child low in iron will be tired, anaemic and possibly a slow learner. Frozen peas are a very good alternative to fresh peas (sadly only available for a few months a year), as they retain most of the nutrients, not to mention a good colour and texture, unlike canned peas.

easy peasy soup

AS ITS NAME SUGGESTS, THIS SOUP COULD BARELY BE EASIER TO MAKE. YOU COULD, OF COURSE, USE FRESH PEAS IF YOU HAVE AN ARMY OF CHILDREN TO HELP POD THEM. I USUALLY DO DOUBLE AND FREEZE SOME. IF USING FRESH PEAS, YOU'LL NEED ABOUT 1.5KG WEIGHT IN THE PODS.

1 tbsp olive oil
1 medium ***onion****, peeled and chopped*
500g podded fresh or frozen ***peas***
750ml vegetable stock
2 tbsp ***mint*** *leaves, roughly chopped*
1 tbsp ***parsley****, roughly chopped*

Heat the olive oil in a large saucepan, add the onion and cook over a medium heat for about 5 minutes until it is soft.

Add the peas and stock, bring to the boil and then turn down the heat to a simmer. Cook for 10 minutes, or until the peas are tender.

Add the mint and parsley and whiz using a hand-held stick blender until you have a fairly smooth soup. Pour into warm bowls and serve.

I usually sprinkle some High five seed mix (page 157) on top of this soup and serve soft brown rolls, spread with tahini, alongside.

traffic light salad

THIS CAN BE EATEN AS A MAIN MEAL IN ITSELF, OR AS A SIDE DISH WITH CHICKEN OR FISH. IT GOES PARTICULARLY WELL WITH CRUNCHY FISH (PAGE 182). IF USING FRESH PEAS, YOU'LL NEED ABOUT 900G WEIGHT IN THE PODS.

2 medium ***sweet potatoes****,*
scrubbed
2 medium ***beetroots****,*
peeled
a little olive oil
300g podded fresh or frozen
peas*, podded*
1 tbsp tamari (or soy sauce)

Preheat the oven to 180°C/Gas 4. Slice the sweet potatoes into 1cm thick rounds and the beetroots into thinner 5mm rounds. Put them into an ovenproof dish, splash with a little olive oil and shake until the discs are all well coated. Roast in the oven for about 30 minutes until they feel tender when pierced with a fork.

Meanwhile, pod fresh peas if using (children can help with this, even little ones). Cook fresh peas in boiling water for 3–5 minutes until barely tender – they should still have a bite. Drain and refresh under running cold water to cool. If using frozen peas, just dunk them in boiling water, then refresh to cool.

When the roasted vegetables are cooked, leave them to cool a little too, then tip into a large dish. Add the peas, drizzle with the tamari and toss to coat, then serve up.

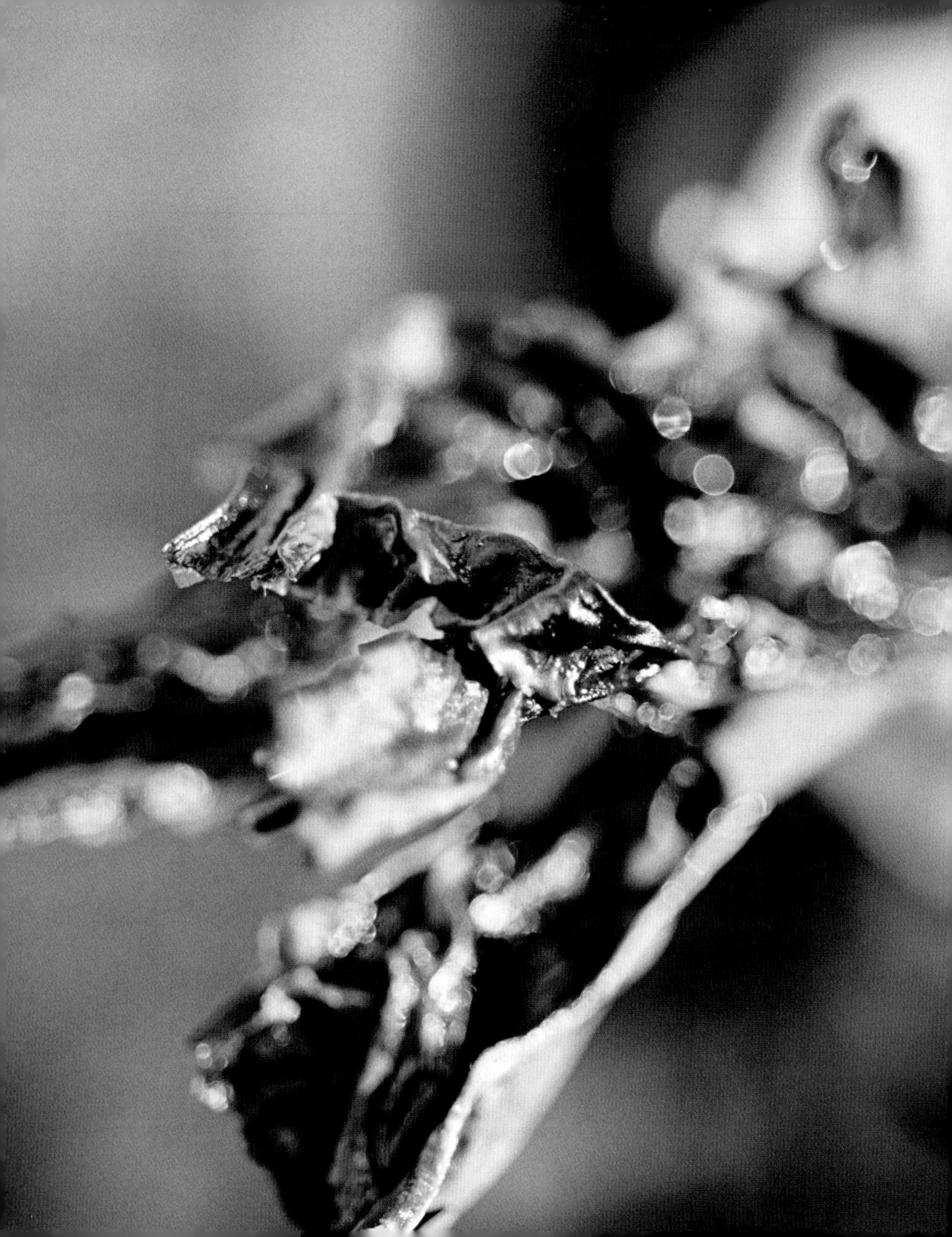

seaweed

You may not be able to get hold of 'fingered tangle' or 'sea otter's cabbage', but there's a whole range of sea vegetables out there that your children could enjoy. For thousands of years, seaweed has been eaten and used medicinally across the world. With their broad spectrum of minerals, like the seawater in which they live, as well as vitamins and other beneficial substances, seaweeds are special wonderfoods. In particular, they are loaded with the mineral iodine, which helps dictate the body's entire metabolism as it is needed to make the thyroid hormone. Seaweed also contains calcium, required for more than just healthy bones, and magnesium, which is important for helping your child cope with any stress that comes along. The folic acid, other B vitamins and iron in seaweed add to its wonderfood value. Other great substances in seaweed are chlorophyll (which makes it green) and alginic acid, both very cleansing and helpful in combating exposure to everyday toxins like lead. Add dried seaweed to soups and stew-like dishes, or rehydrate to use in salads, omelettes and stir-fries.

submarine soup

THIS SOUP IS WONDERFULLY SPEEDY TO MAKE AND IT'S SUBSTANTIAL ENOUGH TO SERVE AS A LIGHT MEAL. YOU COULD USE TOFU INSTEAD OF THE PRAWNS, EVEN IF IT ISN'T A SUBMARINE CREATURE! AND YOU COULD DROP IN SOME NOODLES TO MAKE IT MORE FILLING.

1.2 litres water
4 tbsp ***miso*** *paste*
2 spring ***onions****, trimmed and very finely sliced*
100g ***shiitake mushrooms****, sliced*
16–20 raw prawns, shelled and deveined
handful of dried ***seaweed****, such as hijike, arame or wakame*

TO FINISH
sesame *oil, to drizzle*
coriander *leaves (optional)*
sweet chilli sauce (optional)

Bring the water to the boil in a large saucepan. Scoop out half a mugful, add the miso paste and stir to dissolve, then pour it back into the pan.

Drop in the spring onions, mushrooms, prawns and seaweed and simmer for 5 minutes.

Ladle the soup into warm bowls and drizzle a little sesame oil on top of each portion. For older children or those who fancy it, scatter with some torn coriander leaves and add a small dash of chilli sauce.

seaweed rice balls

IF YOU AND YOUR CHILDREN ARE FAMILIAR WITH IT, FEEL FREE TO USE RAW FISH FOR THESE, PROVIDED IT IS VERY FRESH SASHIMI-GRADE.

*200g **brown rice***
4 tbsp mirin
*½ **cucumber***
*1 **carrot**, peeled*
*200g baked or poached **salmon** or **chicken** fillet*
*8 sheets nori (dried **seaweed**)*
TO SERVE
tamari
Japanese pickled ginger (optional)

Cook the brown rice as directed on the packet, allowing at least 35 minutes to be sure it is tender. Drain if necessary. Tip the rice into a large bowl, stir in the mirin and leave it to cool.

Meanwhile, cut the cucumber and carrot into thin strips. Flake the salmon or shred the chicken. Lay these ingredients and the seaweed on plates.

Get the children to make their own 'sushi'. To do this, take a handful of rice and flatten it in the hand, put some cucumber, carrot and fish or chicken on top and roll the rice around the filling to make a ball. Then wrap it in seaweed – wetting the fingers slightly in a little bowl of water will help to seal the edges of the seaweed. It doesn't really matter what the rolls look like!

Dip the rice balls in a little tamari before each mouthful, which can be eaten with a little pickled ginger if your children like it.

NOTE If you can't get pickled ginger, a lovely dip for the 'sushi' is tamari mixed with a little grated fresh ginger and some sesame oil.

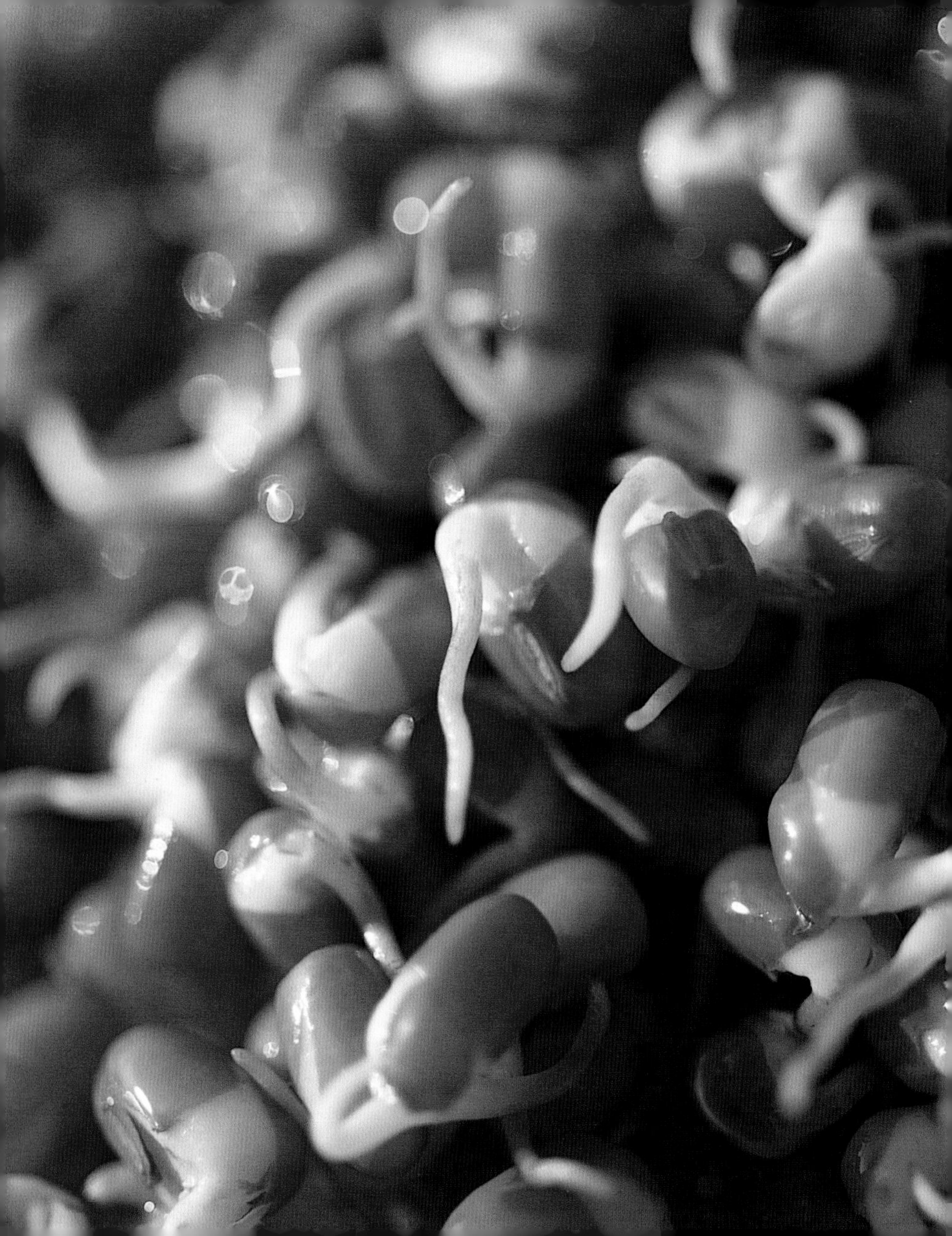

sprouting seeds

This is where you get to indulge in that child-like excitement you may not have felt since getting your fuzzy, cress-ridden cotton wool out of the cupboard. Growing sprouts to eat – from beans, seeds, grains and nuts – is not only simple and fun for children, but also cheap and wonderfully nutritious. Inside a seed is a range of nutrients, waiting to be activated by water in order to sprout and give 'birth' to a whole plant. As the seed absorbs water, the starches, proteins and fats are transformed into much more digestible forms, making it easier for your child's gut to get the most out of them. Some children, who don't react well to certain grains or seeds, are fine when they eat the sprouted versions. What's more, the nutrient density of sprouts is more concentrated than in the grown plants. The particular benefits of each sprout depend on the kind of seed. For example, broccoli seeds contain powerfully cleansing, anti-cancer compounds called glucosinolates, which are even more potent than in broccoli itself, while crunchy mung bean sprouts are a good source of vitamins, minerals and amino acids.

garden in a jar

THIS IS A WONDERFUL WAY TO INTRODUCE CHILDREN TO GROWING THEIR OWN FOOD, IF THEY DON'T ALREADY – AND YOU CAN DO IT WITHOUT SO MUCH AS A BALCONY. LARGE HEALTH FOOD SHOPS SELL SPECIAL TRAYS AND JARS DESIGNED FOR GROWING SPROUTS, BUT THIS IS JUST AS SIMPLE.

about 2 tbsp ***seeds****, such as mung beans, aduki, sunflower, alfalfa, broccoli or radish*

Punch several holes in the screw-top metal lid of a large clean jar, using a skewer. Put your chosen beans or seeds into the jar. Use just one type of seed per jar, as they grow at different rates (mung are a good one to start with). Soak the seeds in plenty of water overnight.

In the morning, tip the jar to drain the water out, rinse the seeds with fresh water and again drain out as much water as possible. Put the jar in a dark cupboard.

Each night and morning, rinse and drain the seeds again until they have sprouted and grown little roots.

After 3–6 days, depending on the seed type and temperature of the cupboard, the sprouts will be tender and edible. If they've developed little leaves, as broccoli and alfalfa sprouts will, place on a windowsill for half a day so the leaves go green.

When they are ready, store the sprouts in the fridge, and use in salads or just as a snack within 3 or 4 days.

wondergreen salad

IF A SALAD IS VARIED IN TASTE AND TEXTURE AND DRESSED WELL, THERE IS NO REASON WHY CHILDREN CANNOT ENJOY IT. YOU CAN OF COURSE, ADD OTHER COLOURS, SUCH AS TOMATOES AND PEPPERS.

3 handfuls of leaves, such as baby ***spinach****, lamb's lettuce and oak leaf lettuce*
2 handfuls of whatever ***sprouts*** *you have, such as mung and alfalfa*
1/3 ***cucumber****, sliced*
1 spring ***onion****, trimmed and finely sliced*
1 firm, ripe ***avocado***
1 tbsp ***pumpkin seeds***
FOR THE DRESSING
1 tsp Dijon mustard
1 small ***garlic*** *clove, peeled and crushed*
1 tbsp cider vinegar or balsamic vinegar
3 tbsp olive oil
ground sea salt
freshly ground black pepper

In a salad bowl, toss all the salad leaves together with the sprouts, cucumber and spring onion.

For the dressing, shake the mustard, garlic and vinegar together in a screw-topped jar, then add the olive oil, salt and pepper and shake again.

Just before serving, halve, stone and peel the avocado, then chop roughly and add to the salad bowl. Drizzle with the dressing and toss to mix, then sprinkle with the pumpkin seeds.

Serve the salad alongside a main course, such as Popeye puffs (page 23) or Dusted drumsticks (page 72).

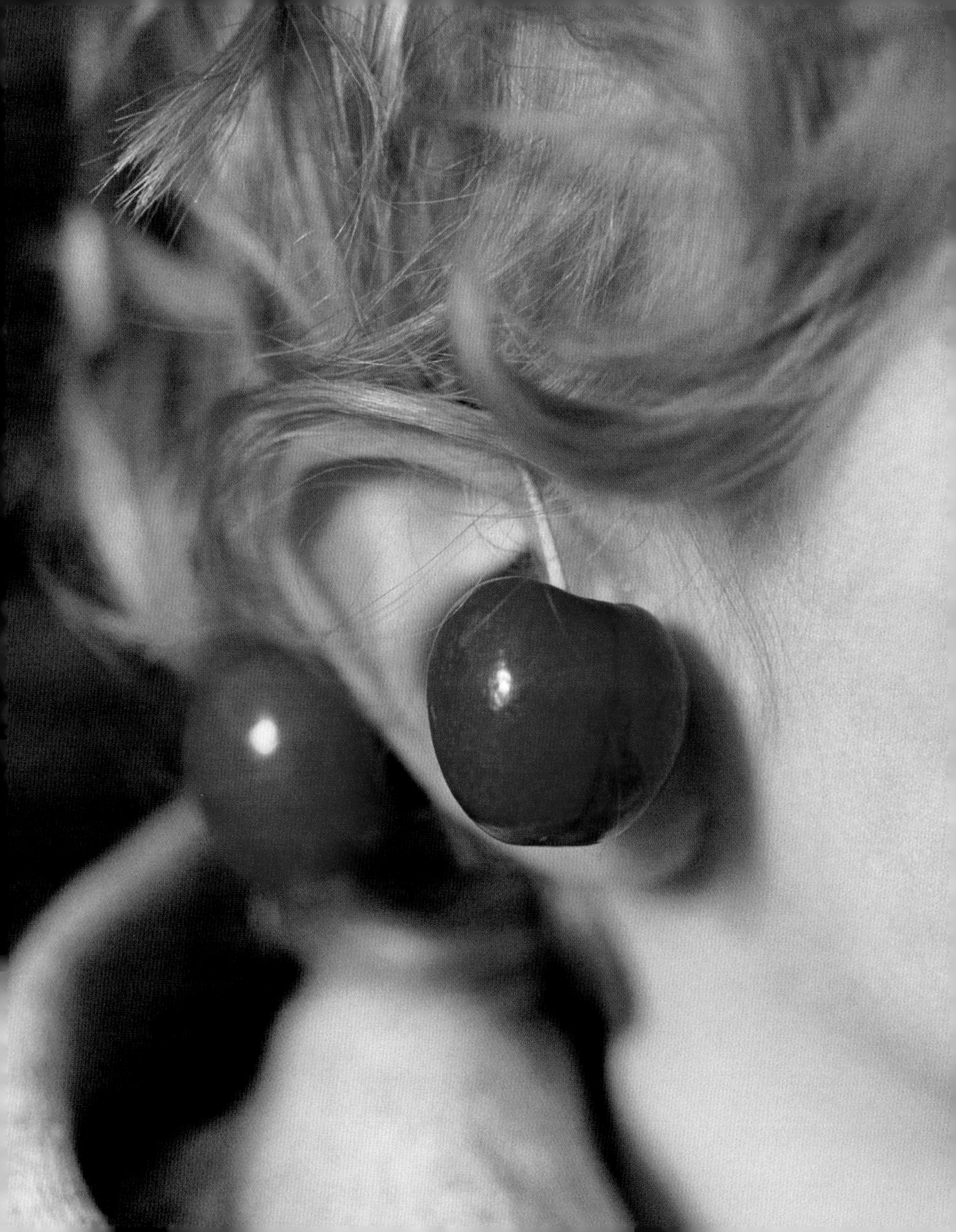

cherries

Eating cherries in my childhood is synonymous with wearing cherry 'earrings', made by hooking double-stalked cherries, one in front and one behind the ear! The fun comes loaded with edible goodness too. Cherries are a wonderful source of healthy sugars for providing energy, but also fibre for keeping the digestive tract in working order. They contain the B vitamin, folic acid, which is essential for growth, plus some iron, beta carotene, vitamin C and small amounts of other micronutrients. Cherries' rich colour points to their content of flavonoids, powerful antioxidants such as anthocyanins and quercetin, that can help quell children's allergic reactions and inflammation and have even shown anti-carcinogenic qualities. They work with vitamin C to boost the body's defence mechanisms and strengthen our 'cellular glue', collagen. The darker the cherries, the higher their anthocyanin and therefore their antioxidant content. In folk medicine, cherries and their juice have been used for treating urinary tract infections and stimulating the body's digestive and detoxification processes for centuries.

grilled lamb in cherry sauce

YOU CAN USE FROZEN OR CANNED, UNSWEETENED PITTED CHERRIES IF YOU CAN'T GET HOLD OF FRESH ONES FOR THIS DISH.

1 tsp olive oil
½ ***onion****, peeled and sliced*
4 star anise
8 small ***lamb*** *chops*
2 tbsp tamari (or soy sauce)
juice of 1 ***orange***
1cm piece fresh root ***ginger****, peeled and grated*
100ml water (or red wine!)
300g ***cherries****, pitted*

Heat the olive oil in a saucepan and soften the onion with the star anise over a medium heat for a few minutes. Brown the lamb chops in the pan (in two batches) for a couple of minutes on each side, then remove them and set aside. Preheat the grill.

Add the tamari, orange juice, ginger and water to the pan and stir well, then add the cherries and bring to the boil. Let bubble for 4–5 minutes, then turn the heat right down and leave to simmer, covered, while you finish the chops.

Grill the chops for about 4 minutes on each side until cooked through.

Serve the chops topped with the cherry sauce and accompanied by boiled buckwheat, quinoa or brown rice and green veg.

cherry 'flan'

THIS IS A VARIATION OF A SPANISH *FLAN* – A SORT OF BAKED CUSTARD. YOU COULD USE FROZEN OR CANNED, UNSWEETENED CHERRIES AND ADD OTHER FRUITS TOO.

300g ***cherries****, pitted*
60g ***buckwheat*** *or wholemeal flour*
60g brown sugar
2 medium ***eggs***
1/2 tsp grated ***lemon*** *zest*
1/2 tsp ground ***cinnamon***
1 tsp vanilla extract
350ml milk or ***soya*** *milk*

Preheat the oven to 190°C/Gas 5. Lightly oil a 23cm flan dish and lay the cherries evenly over the bottom (younger children can do this).

Using a hand-held stick blender, mix the flour, sugar, eggs, lemon zest, cinnamon, vanilla extract and milk together until smooth.

Carefully pour the custard over the cherries and bake in the oven for about 45 minutes until the custard is set. To test, insert a fine skewer or knife tip into the centre – it should come out clean. Serve warm.

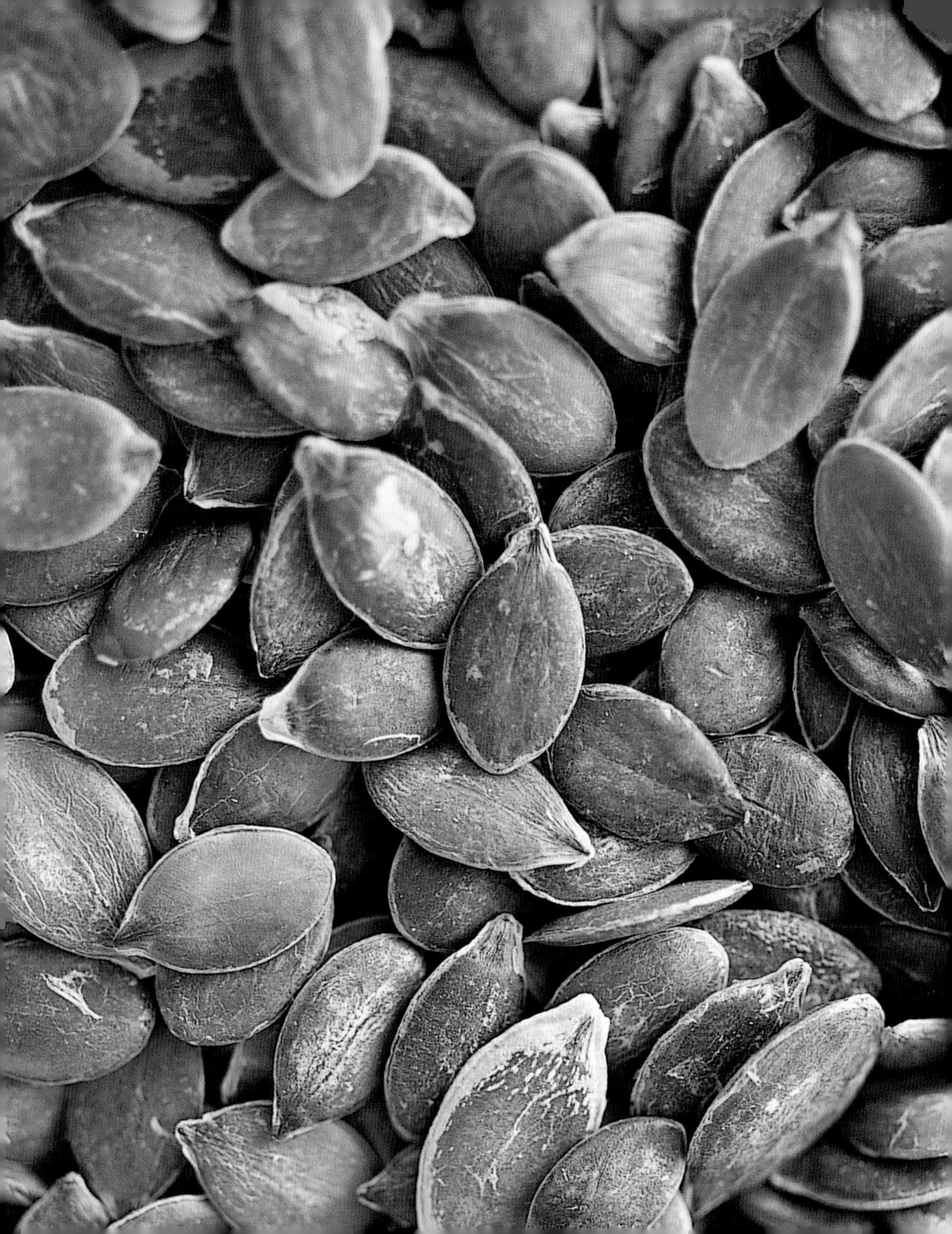

pumpkin seeds

A more reliable source of these packages of goodness, if you don't scoop them from a Hallowe'en pumpkin, is a healthfood shop. These green seeds are tiny powerhouses of a wide range of vital nutrients for development and repair in growing little people. They are particularly rich in zinc and vitamin B_6, which are needed for proper growth, immunity, sexual development and clear skin. And their calcium and magnesium are vital for healthy bone building, strong teeth, nerve firing, muscle contraction and relaxation. The essential fatty acids (EFAs) in pumpkin seeds are a star feature. These EFAs are important for smooth skin and their anti-inflammatory properties, both of which are useful for children with dry skin or eczema. EFAs are incorporated into every cell membrane. When cell membranes are healthy, it means that cells communicate properly and 'hear' hormonal messages that dictate metabolism, hormone balance, mood and much more. Pumpkin seeds contribute a good source of protein to the diets of vegetarian and vegan children; their fat and protein make them a satisfying snack.

speckled porridge

THIS IS A GREAT WAY TO SEND THE CHILDREN OFF TO SCHOOL SO THEIR ENERGY AND CONCENTRATION ARE OPTIMISED FOR THE MORNING. INSTEAD OF APPLE, YOU COULD ADD A COUPLE OF SPOONFULS OF FRUIT COMPOTE (PAGE 217) IF YOU LIKE.
SERVES 2

4 tbsp porridge ***oats***
milk or ***soya*** *milk (about 200ml)*
1 ***apple****, grated*
1 tsp ***honey***
1 tbsp ***pumpkin seeds*** *or* ***High five seed mix*** *(page 157)*

Put the oats into a saucepan, add enough water to cover and stir gently with a wooden spoon over a low heat. As the oats begin to absorb the water, slowly start to add the milk, stirring continuously, then add the apple. Each time the porridge starts to thicken, add a little more milk to keep it slightly runny.

When the oats are cooked – this should take about 5 minutes – stir in the honey. Top with the pumpkin seeds or High five seed mix and serve.

chewy flapjacks

THESE MAKE A DELICIOUS, ENERGY-FILLED TEATIME SNACK OR LUNCHBOX TREAT.

150g porridge ***oats***
75g puffed ***rice***, ***quinoa*** *and/or wheat flakes*
100g ***raisins*** *and/or other dried fruit, such as* ***apple*** *or* ***peach***
50g dried ***apricots***, *chopped to raisin size*
50g ***pumpkin seeds***
50g butter
3 tbsp ***honey***
2 ***egg*** *whites*
175ml ***apple*** *juice*

Preheat the oven to 180°C/Gas 4. Lightly oil a shallow baking tin, about 30 x 20cm, or line it with greaseproof paper. In a large bowl, mix the oats, puffed cereal, raisins, chopped apricots and pumpkin seeds together.

In a small saucepan over a low heat, gently melt the butter with the honey until it is very runny (do not let it boil). Pour the melted mixture on to the oat mix, then add the egg whites and apple juice. Mix thoroughly until evenly combined.

Press the moist cereal into the baking tin and bake in the oven for 20–25 minutes. Leave to cool in the tin, then turn out and cut into bars. Store in an airtight container for up to 5 days.

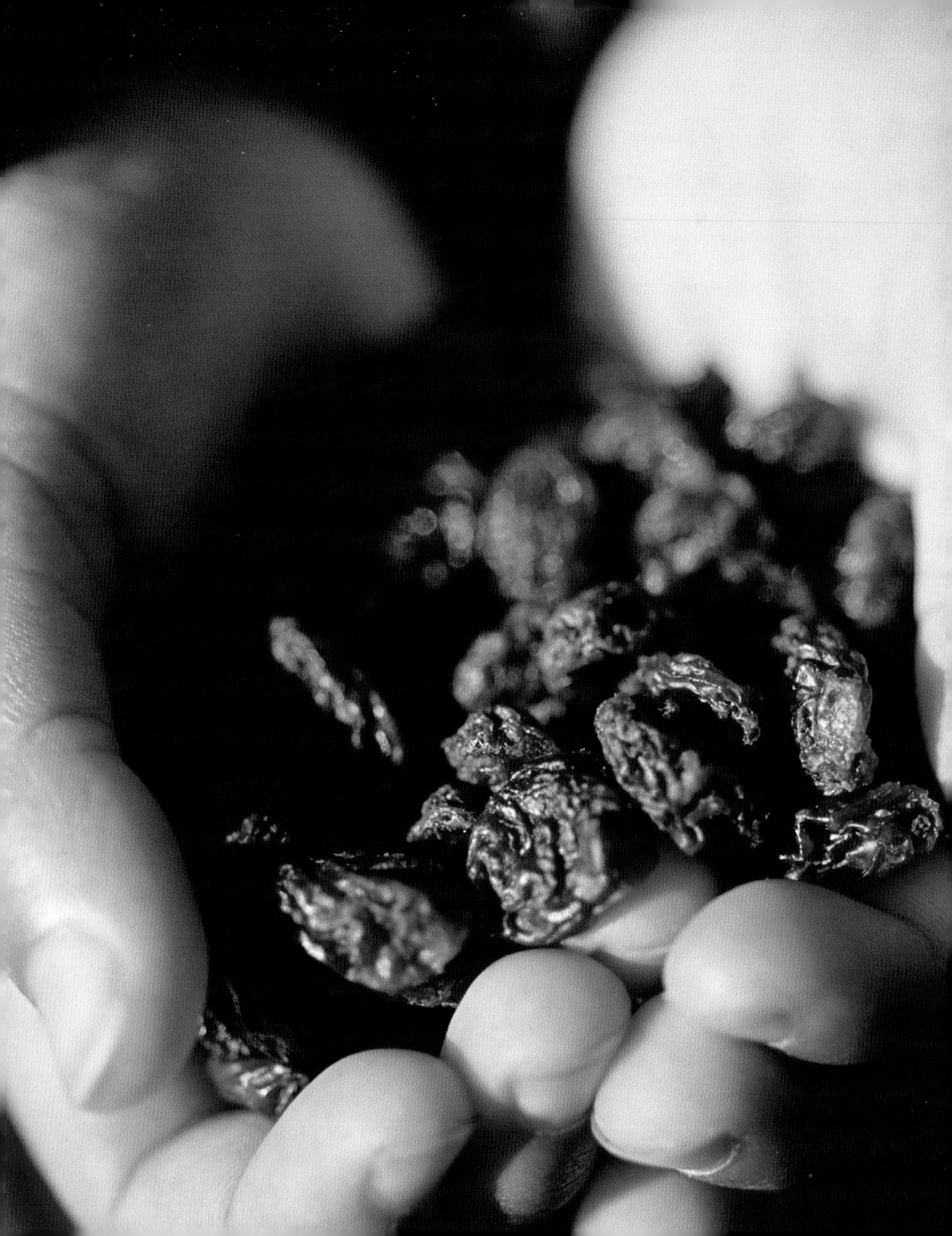

raisins

Probably one of children's favourite 'health' foods, it's not hard to see why raisins are so appealing; they're sweet, easy to eat, easily transportable and don't make a mess. Similar to grapes, their original form, raisins are loaded with key antioxidants such as those in the phenol family, though some are lost in the dehydration process. Natural chemicals such as procyanidins offer children protection against pollution and illness. Raisins contain a range of vitamins and minerals, particularly iron and potassium, and they are virtually fat free. As any child who has overdosed on raisins will know, they can cause bloating and wind. In small quantities though, their fibre is very useful in cleansing the gut and preventing constipation. Raisins are a condensed source of natural sugars, which are good for boosting energy, especially as they come 'packaged' with so much other goodness. Scientists have isolated phytonutrients in raisins, such as oleanolic acid, which fight the bacteria in the mouth that cause cavities and gum disease, so the effect of the sugar content of raisins on teeth isn't quite so much of a worry.

pink & green kedgeree

OK, SO THIS ISN'T REALLY A KEDGEREE AT ALL, BUT IT IS FISH WITH RICE AND COLOURFUL VEG, WHICH NOT ONLY MAKE IT MORE APPEALING TO THE EYE BUT ALSO ADD GOODNESS. YOU CAN DO A LUXURY VERSION WITH SMOKED SALMON IN PLACE OF HADDOCK IF YOU LIKE.

200g ***brown rice***
200g ***haddock*** *fillet*
200g undyed, smoked ***haddock*** *fillet*
2 medium ***tomatoes***
splash of olive oil
knob of butter
1 ***onion****, peeled and finely diced*
3 tbsp ***raisins***
100g frozen ***peas***

Cook the brown rice as directed on the packet, allowing at least 35 minutes to be sure it is tender. Meanwhile, cut the fresh and smoked fish into cubes, checking for any small bones. Immerse the tomatoes in a pan of boiling water for a minute to loosen the skins, then remove and peel when cool enough to handle. Roughly chop the tomato flesh.

Heat the olive oil and butter in a large pan and gently cook the onion with the raisins for at least 5 minutes, without letting the onion brown too much. Add the fish cubes, tomatoes and peas and cook, stirring occasionally, for 4–5 minutes until the fish is cooked through.

When the rice is tender, drain if necessary and add it to the fish mix. Stir it all together and serve with a salad, such as Baby greens with raspberries (page 56).

crunchy cookies

THIS QUANTITY MAKES ABOUT 20 VERY HEALTHY AND DELICIOUS BISCUITS.

100g porridge ***oats***
125g wholemeal flour
30g brown sugar
1½ tsp ground ***cinnamon***
75g ***raisins***
1 tbsp ***sunflower seeds***
2 tbsp ***sesame seeds***
1 medium ***egg***
2 tbsp melted butter
6 tbsp milk or ***soya*** *milk*

Preheat the oven to 180°C/Gas 4. Line two large baking sheets with non-stick baking paper. Finely grind the oats in a blender, then tip into a mixing bowl. Add the flour, sugar, cinnamon, raisins and seeds and stir until evenly mixed.

Beat the egg in another bowl and mix in the melted butter and milk. Pour on to the dry ingredients and mix well to combine.

Spoon walnut-sized balls of the mixture on to the lined trays, spacing well apart, and flatten them into rough cookie shapes. Bake in the oven for about 15 minutes, watching carefully to make sure they don't overcook.

Leave the cookies on the baking sheets for a few minutes to firm up. Then transfer to a wire rack to cool. Store any that aren't eaten straight away in an airtight container for up to 5 days.

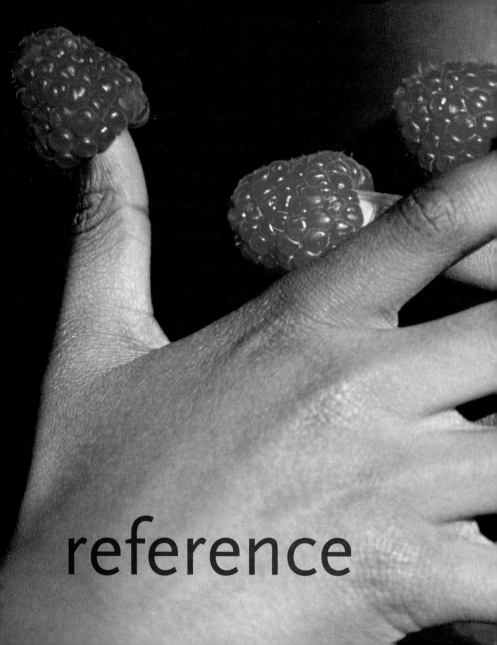

reference

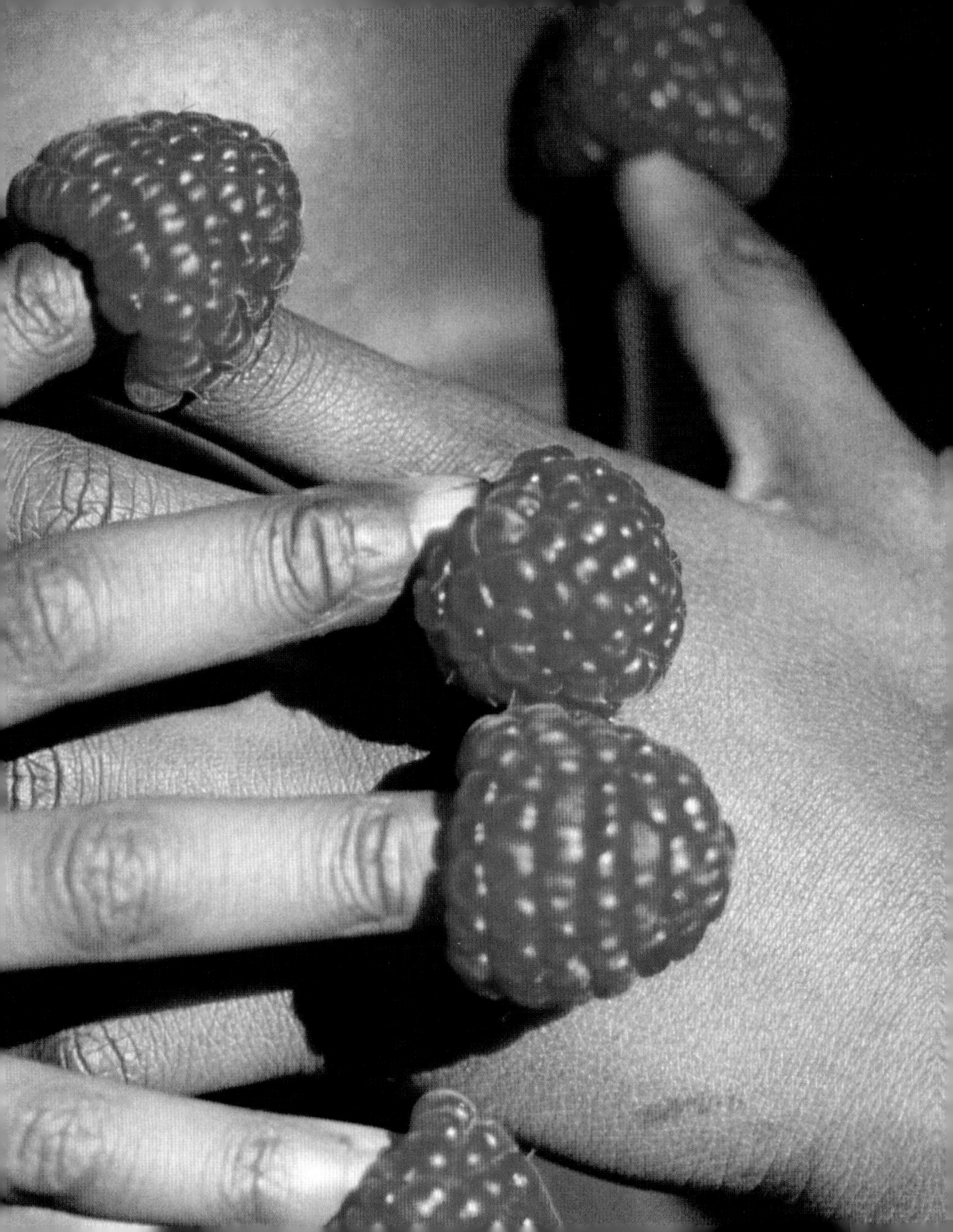

wonderfoods week

YOU COULD FEED YOUR CHILDREN EVERY MEAL ON WONDERFOOD-PACKED RECIPES. HERE'S A SAMPLE WEEK TO SHOW YOU HOW. DEPENDING ON THE AGE OF YOUR CHILD AND HIS/HER APPETITE, YOU MAY NEED TO ADD TO THIS, FOR EXAMPLE A SMOOTHIE AND/OR A BOWL OF CEREAL FOR A BIGGER BREAKFAST. IF YOUR CHILD IS AT SCHOOL AND TAKES A PACKED LUNCH, SIMPLY REPLACE THE LUNCHES SUGGESTED BELOW WITH PACKED LUNCHES FROM THE IDEAS LISTED OPPOSITE.

	Breakfast	***Lunch***	***Main Meal***	***Dessert/Teatime***
Mon	*Tropical smoothie (page 26)*	*Vampire pâté sandwich (page 254)*	*Salmon satay (page 171)*	*Chocolate apples (page 41)*
Tues	*Monster chomp cereal (page 195)*	*Pineapple boats (page 68)*	*Chickpea & coconut curry (page 90)*	*Raspberry brûlée (page 57)*
Wed	*Fresh fruit & ginger soup (page 76)*	*Baked veggies on toast (page 226)*	*Grilled lamb in cherry sauce (page 288)*	*Fruit compote (page 217)*
Thurs	*Speckled porridge (page 292)*	*Avocado dip & chips (page 178)*	*Sticky chicken (page 153)*	*Coconut rice pud with nectarines (page 122)*
Fri	*Juicy fruits (page 73)*	*Easy peasy soup (page 276)*	*Mini fish & chips (page 266)*	*Kiwi lollies (page 238)*
Sat	*Black banana pancakes (page 216)*	*Buckwheat salad (page 111)*	*Mushroom slice (page 225)*	*Cherry 'flan' (page 289)*
Sun	*Super scrambled eggs (page 160)*	*Jacket potato with Sweet purple filling (page 44)*	*Lemon roast chicken (page 221)*	*Griddled apple rings (page 65)*

wonderfoods packed lunches

MANY PARENTS FIND THAT EVEN IF THEY GIVE THEIR CHILDREN GOOD QUALITY, HEALTHY FOODS AT HOME, IT'S A DIFFERENT MATTER AS SOON AS THE CHILDREN ARE OUT OF THE DOOR. KEEPING PACKED LUNCHES HEALTHY AND VARIED CAN BE QUITE A CHALLENGE – IT'S ALL TOO EASY TO RELY ON THE SAME SANDWICHES, CRISPS AND A SWEET BAR OF SOMETHING. HERE'S TWO WEEK'S WORTH OF IDEAS FROM RECIPES IN THE BOOK THAT CAN SERVE AS FRESH INSPIRATION FOR YOUR CHILDREN'S LUNCHBOXES.

Main	***Dessert***
Butternut soup (page 30) with bread	*Crunchy cookies (page 297)*
Dusted drumsticks (page 72), Spiced quinoa (page 167) and cherry tomatoes	*Chewy flapjacks (page 293)*
Edible spoons (page 106), Chickpea dip (page 89) and crackers	*Apricot crunch clusters (page 251)*
Pear & Parma rolls (page 102) and rye bread spread with tahini	*Apple custard slice (page 163)*
Stop-go slice (page 161)	*Rainbow fruit salad (page 239)*
Ham & Puy salad (page 179)	*Blubbery fool (page 247)*
Turkey balls (page 258) in pitta bread with Chickpea dip (page 89)	*Fruit compote (page 217)*
Big tomato sandwich (page 206)	*Pineapple lassi (page 144)*
Green & white salad (page 136) and crackers	*Peach slice (page 123)*
Seaweed rice balls (page 281)	*Banana passion pots (page 18)*

wonderfoods nutrient sources

CHILDREN NEED A BROAD RANGE OF NUTRIENTS FROM THEIR DIET IN ORDER TO GROW AND DEVELOP PROPERLY, AND TO STAY WELL. HERE IS AN OUTLINE OF THE KEY NUTRIENTS, THEIR ROLES IN THE BODY AND THE WONDERFOODS YOUR CHILD CAN EAT TO GET THEM.

Nutrient	Nutrient for...
Protein	Proteins are molecules made up of amino acids linked together in a particular order specified by a gene. They are needed for the structure, function and regulation of all the body's cells and organs. Hormones, neurotransmitters, enzymes, transporters and immune cells are proteins.
Carbohydrate	These are sugars and starches that the body breaks down into glucose, a simple sugar used by the body as fuel for its cells to make energy. They are found in sugar, cereals, the wonderfoods listed opposite and other foods. The body also uses carbohydrate to make a substance called glycogen, which is stored in the liver and muscles for future use.
Unsaturated Fat	These fats are an essential part of a child's diet as they provide essential fatty acids (EFAs) that the body cannot produce itself. They are needed for effectively functioning cell membranes i.e. so every cell can do its job well; healthy nerve and brain activities; smooth skin; good hormone balance; cardiovascular health (blood that is not too 'sticky', flexible blood vessels); and they have anti-inflammatory properties.
Saturated Fat	Often labelled the 'bad fats', saturated fats, in moderate quantities are a perfectly valid part of any varied diet. Not only are they a source of energy but they also help the body to absorb some vitamins. Foods containing saturated fats are also excellent sources of other nutrients e.g. meat for protein or yoghurt for calcium. In excessive amounts, they have been linked to heart disease and obesity.

Wonderfood sources

Egg, fish, turkey, chicken, lamb, yoghurt, soya, nuts, seeds, beans, lentils
All fruit and vegetables, rice, buckwheat, oats, quinoa, rye, sweet potatoes, lentils , beans, honey
Fish, seeds, nuts, olive oil
Butter, yoghurt, milk, cheese, meat

Vitamin	Nutrient for...
Vitamin A/beta carotene	Antioxidant; protects skin and 'internal skin' – lungs, gut; eyes; immunity
Vitamin B1	Energy production; nervous system; carbohydrate processing
Vitamin B2	Energy; skin; nervous system
Vitamin B3	Energy; nervous system; moods; blood sugar balance; stress response; hormone balance
Vitamin B5	Energy production; stress response; regeneration of cells; anti-inflammatory; immunity
Vitamin B6	Energy production; nervous system; moods and brain power; hormone balance; protein digestion; immunity
Vitamin B12	Brain and nervous system; red blood cell formation; cellular energy and reproduction; works with folic acid
Folic Acid	Brain and nervous system, especially in foetal growth; cellular energy and reproduction; moods; cardiovascular health; red blood cell formation
Biotin	Energy production; fat and amino acid processing; skin, nails and hair
Vitamin C	Antioxidant; collagen formation: skin, blood vessels and gums; aids iron absorption; immunity; helps protect against illness, allergies, pollution and stress; anti-inflammatory
Vitamin D	Helps calcium usage; bones and teeth; some cancer protection
Vitamin E	Antioxidant; immunity; helps protect skin, brain, circulation and hormones; cardiovascular system
Vitamin K	Blood clotting; bone building

Wonderfood sources

Apricots, broccoli, carrot, pumpkin, spinach, sweet potato, melon, watermelon, egg

Beans, sunflower seeds, fish, brown rice, oats, rye, quinoa, buckwheat, chicken, turkey, lamb, egg

Nuts, oats, spinach, yoghurt, egg, fish, chicken, turkey, lamb

Chicken, turkey, lamb, fish, seeds, beans, lentils, soya, yoghurt

Egg, fish, chicken, turkey, lamb, brown rice, oats, rye, quinoa, buckwheat, lentils, soya

Chicken, turkey, fish, lamb, nuts, brown rice, oats, rye, quinoa, buckwheat, avocado, bananas, seeds, beans, lentils

Egg, fish, chicken, turkey, lamb, yoghurt

All fruits, beans, lentils, soya, spinach, parsley, oats, rye, quinoa, buckwheat

Egg, brown rice, oats, rye, quinoa, buckwheat, lentils, fish, seeds

Blackcurrants, berries, broccoli, cabbage, lemon, lime, orange, sweet pepper, kiwi fruit, spinach, tomatoes

Fish, egg, yoghurt

Nuts, seeds and seed oils, egg

Sprouts, green beans, parsley, spinach, broccoli

Mineral	Nutrient for...
Calcium	Bone building; muscle contraction and relaxation; regular heart beat; blood clotting; nerve transmission
Chromium	Processing of carbohydrates and sugars; blood sugar balance; works with insulin
Copper	Production and transport of red blood cells; iron absorption; antioxidant
Iodine	Forms part of thyroid hormone
Iron	Forms part of haemoglobin i.e. helps transport oxygen; other uses include cell reproduction
Magnesium	Energy production; hormone balance; muscle and nerve function; cardiovascular health; blood sugar balance; works with calcium
Manganese	Antioxidant; energy production; nerves and brain; blood sugar balance
Potassium	Works with sodium to control fluid balance; blood pressure, nerves, muscles
Selenium	Antioxidant; works with vitamin E; immunity; cardiovascular health; anti-inflammatory
Sulphur	Antioxidant; helps liver detoxification; collagen production; skin, hair, nails
Zinc	Antioxidant; growth and development; all protein production; energy production; hormone production and balance; digestion; skin health

Wonderfood sources

Nuts, seeds, spinach, broccoli, canned fish, yoghurt

Chicken, turkey, lamb, egg, fish, brown rice, oats, rye, quinoa, buckwheat, nuts, sweet pepper

Fish, nuts, seeds, oats, rye, quinoa, buckwheat

Fish, seaweed

Egg, chicken, turkey, lamb, fish, seeds, seaweed, spinach, brown rice, oats, rye, quinoa, buckwheat

Brown rice, oats, rye, quinoa, buckwheat, seeds, nuts

Avocado, berries, buckwheat, ginger, nuts, oats, seaweed, spinach

Avocado, banana, lemon, lime, orange fruit, lentils, nuts, spinach, whole grains, cherries

Fish, seeds, brown rice, oats, rye, quinoa, buckwheat, nuts

Cabbage, egg, fish, garlic, onions

Egg, fish, chicken, turkey, lamb, seeds, yoghurt

wonderfoods therapy

FOR CHILDREN TO KEEP FIT AND WELL, THEY NEED TO HAVE A BROAD RANGE OF FOODS, BUT THERE ARE CERTAIN ONES THAT CAN HELP BOOST THE BODY TO LIMIT THE CHANCES OF AN ILLNESS OR CONDITION TAKING HOLD. THAT SAID, IF YOUR CHILD DOES SUCCUMB, CERTAIN FOODS CAN HELP SUPPORT THE BODY AT TIMES OF ILLNESS TO RELIEVE THE SYMPTOMS AND ENCOURAGE HEALING. GIVING YOUR CHILD THE FOODS SUGGESTED IS NOT INTENDED AS A REPLACEMENT FOR MEDICAL ADVICE.

	Wonderfoods to eat
Acne	*All fruit and vegetable fibre, oats, rye, brown rice, beans, lentils, beetroot, greens e.g. spinach, broccoli, parsley, avocado, nuts, strawberries, mango, pumpkin, sweet potato, carrot, garlic, seeds, yoghurt*
ADHD	*Seeds and seed oils, oily fish, yoghurt, turkey, chicken, egg, nuts, all fresh fruit and vegetables, oats, rye, quinoa, brown rice, beans, lentils*
Anaemia	*Greens e.g. spinach, broccoli, parsley, beetroot, strawberries, kiwi fruit, orange, lemon, lime, lamb, fish, egg, turkey, chicken*
Asthma	*All fresh fruit and vegetables especially berries, blackcurrants and cherries, carrot, sweet pepper, apricot, peach, nectarine, broccoli, ginger, garlic, seeds and seed oils, oily fish, onion, nuts, pumpkin, sweet potato*
Behavioural problems	*Seeds and seed oils, oily fish, yoghurt, turkey, chicken, egg, nuts, all fresh fruit and vegetables, oats, rye, quinoa, brown rice, beans, lentils*
Bronchitis	*Apricot, sweet pepper, cherries, watermelon, melon, blackcurrants, peach, nectarine, broccoli, strawberries, kiwi fruit, orange, lemon, lime, garlic, seeds, pumpkin, sweet potato, onion, shiitake mushrooms, cinnamon, cloves*
Burns, cuts & bruises	*Apricot, sweet pepper, carrot, peach, nectarine, cherries, watermelon, melon, broccoli, strawberries, kiwi fruit, orange, lemon, lime, garlic, seeds, avocado, nuts, mango, pumpkin, sweet potato*

Chickenpox	*Berries, cherries, watermelon, melon, broccoli, blackcurrants, strawberries, kiwi fruit, orange, lemon, lime, garlic, carrot, sweet pepper, apricot, mango, avocado, pumpkin, sweet potato, seeds, garlic, oily fish*
Chronic fatigue	*Greens e.g. spinach, broccoli, parsley, strawberries, kiwi fruit, orange, lemon, lime, yoghurt, lamb, egg, turkey, chicken, seeds and seed oils, fish, oats, seaweed, buckwheat*
Cold Sores	*Berries, cherries, watermelon, melon, broccoli, blackcurrants, strawberries, kiwi fruit, orange, lemon, lime, garlic, carrot, sweet pepper, apricot, avocado, mango, pumpkin, sweet potato, shiitake mushrooms, oily fish*
Colitis	*Berries, watermelon, melon, broccoli, blackcurrants, strawberries, kiwi fruit, garlic, carrot, sweet pepper, apricot, pineapple, seeds and seed oils, oily fish, turmeric, cardamom*
Common cold & flu	*All fresh fruit and vegetables especially berries, blackcurrants, carrot, apricot, broccoli, strawberries, kiwi fruit, pumpkin, sweet potato, garlic, onion, ginger, pineapple, seeds and seed oils, cloves, cinnamon*
Constipation	*All fruit and vegetables, oats, rye, brown rice, beans, lentils, seeds and seed oils, plenty of water and vegetable juices, beetroot, cucumber*
Coughs	*Apricot, sweet pepper, cherries, watermelon, melon, peach, nectarine, blackcurrants, broccoli, strawberries, kiwi fruit, orange, lemon, lime, garlic, seeds, pumpkin, sweet potato, onion, shiitake mushrooms, cinnamon, cloves*
Dermatitis	*All fresh fruit and vegetables especially berries, carrot, sweet pepper, apricot, peach, nectarine, broccoli, avocado, nuts, mango, pumpkin, sweet potato, ginger, garlic, seeds and seed oils, oily fish*
Diabetes	*All fruit and vegetable fibre, oats, rye, brown rice, beans, lentils, greens e.g. spinach, broccoli, parsley, yoghurt, egg, turkey, chicken, seeds and seed oils, fish*
Diarrhoea	*Apple, carrot (cooked), white rice, plenty of water, yoghurt*

Dry skin	*Berries, watermelon, melon, peach, nectarine, broccoli, kiwi fruit, garlic, carrot, sweet peppers, apricot, avocado, nuts, mango, seeds and seed oils, oily fish*
Ear infection	*Berries, broccoli, blackcurrants, strawberries, kiwi fruit, orange, lemon, lime, garlic, onion, ginger, sweet potato, carrot, sweet pepper, apricot, seeds and seed oils*
Eczema	*Berries, cherries, carrot, sweet pepper, apricot, peach, nectarine, broccoli, avocado, nuts, mango, pumpkin, sweet potato, ginger, garlic, seeds and seed oils, oily fish, turmeric, nuts*
Fever	*Fresh fruit and vegetable juices, berries, blackcurrants, broccoli, kiwi fruit, strawberries, orange, lemon, lime, garlic, carrot, sweet pepper, shiitake mushrooms, apricot*
Hay fever	*All fresh fruit and vegetables especially berries, cherries and blackcurrants, carrot, sweet pepper, apricot, broccoli, ginger, garlic, seeds and seed oils, oily fish*
Hives	*All fresh fruit and vegetables especially berries, carrot, sweet pepper, apricot, peach, nectarine, broccoli, avocado, nuts, mango, pumpkin, sweet potato, ginger, garlic, seeds and seed oils, oily fish*
Hyperactivity	*Seeds and seed oils, oily fish, yoghurt, turkey, chicken, egg, nuts, all fresh fruit and vegetables, oats, rye, quinoa, brown rice, beans, lentils*
Impetigo	*Berries, blackcurrants, watermelon, peach, nectarine, melon, broccoli, kiwi fruit, strawberries, orange, lemon, lime, garlic, spinach, carrot, parsley, beetroot, avocado, cucumber, shiitake mushrooms, mango, pumpkin, sweet potato*
Irritable bowel syndrome	*Pineapple, cabbage, fresh vegetable juices, spinach, broccoli, parsley, yoghurt, garlic, onion, ginger, cardamom, pineapple, cucumber*
Learning difficulties	*Seeds and seed oils, oily fish, thyme, egg, berries, watermelon, melon, blackcurrants, broccoli, strawberries, kiwi fruit, orange, lemon, lime, turmeric, nuts*

Mumps	*Berries, cherries, watermelon, melon, broccoli, blackcurrants, strawberries, kiwi fruit, orange, lemon, lime, garlic, carrot, sweet pepper, apricot, avocado, mango, pumpkin, sweet potato, shiitake mushrooms, oily fish*
Period problems	*All fruit and vegetable fibre, oats, rye, brown rice, beans, lentils, greens e.g. spinach, broccoli, parsley, soya, seeds and seed oils, oily fish, seaweed*
Psoriasis	*Berries, carrot, pepper, apricot, peach, nectarine, cherries, broccoli, avocado, nuts, mango, pumpkin, sweet potato, ginger, garlic, seeds and seed oils, oily fish, turmeric*
Sinusitis	*All fresh fruit and vegetables especially berries and blackcurrants, carrot, apricot, broccoli, strawberries, kiwi fruit, garlic, onion, ginger, pineapple, shiitake mushrooms, seeds and seed oils*
Sleeping problems	*Spinach, broccoli, parsley, yoghurt, chicken, turkey, seeds, buckwheat, oats*
Sprains, strains & other injuries	*Spinach, broccoli, parsley, seeds, garlic, cherries, pineapple, seeds and seed oils*
Stress	*Yoghurt, egg, turkey, chicken, lamb, seeds and seed oils, fish, spinach, broccoli, parsley, strawberries, kiwi fruit, orange, lemon, lime, oats, quinoa, rye*
Tonsillitis	*Berries, broccoli, blackcurrants, cherries, strawberries, kiwi fruit, orange, lemon, lime, garlic, onion, ginger, sweet potato, carrot, sweet pepper, apricot, seeds and seed oils, shiitake mushrooms*
Travel sickness	*Ginger, cardamom, cinnamon*
Verrucas	*Berries, cherries, watermelon, melon, broccoli, blackcurrants, strawberries, kiwi fruit, orange, lemon, lime, garlic, carrot, sweet pepper, apricot, avocado, mango, pumpkin, sweet potato, shiitake mushrooms, oily fish*
Warts	*Berries, cherries, watermelon, melon, broccoli, blackcurrants, strawberries, kiwi fruit, orange, lemon, lime, garlic, carrot, sweet pepper, apricot, avocado, mango, pumpkin, sweet potato, shiitake mushrooms, oily fish*

wonderfoods glossary

amino acid The building blocks of proteins in our food and throughout the body.

anthocyanidins Powerful antioxidant chemicals found in some plants, particularly blue, red and purple ones.

antihistamine A substance that counteracts the action of the inflammatory, allergic body chemical histamine.

antioxidant A substance or enzyme that neutralises oxidants, or free radicals, protecting cells from damage that can lead to disease and ageing.

bacteria Minute, single-celled organisms that live in us and in the environment. Some are harmful and others are beneficial.

bioflavonoids Antioxidant chemicals found in some foods.

carotenoids A family of colourful compounds found in foods with antioxidant properties that are considered to be plant forms of vitamin A.

chlorophyll The green pigment in plants, which they need to capture sunlight in order to produce energy.

cholesterol A fat-like substance found in some foods, produced in the liver and present throughout the human body. It's needed in the body, in cell structure for example, and for making some hormones. In excess, it can be a harmful component of cardiovascular disease, particularly when oxidised.

complex carbohydrate Starches and fibre in foods that have not been refined; the starches can be broken down to produce energy.

detoxification The body's natural 'cleansing' processes by which it clears waste products and eliminates them.

diuretic A substance that increases urination, promoting water loss from the body.

enzyme A protein that acts as a catalyst in any of the countless processes in the body. The term also describes substances that help the breakdown of foods in the gut.

essential fatty acids (EFAs) Fats, such as those found in fish, nuts and seeds, that are a necessary part of our diet for good health.

fibre A part of foods, especially fruit, vegetables and whole grains, that the gut can't digest. Fibre helps slow down the release of digested food as glucose into the bloodstream, bulks out the stool, feeds beneficial bacteria and encourages the elimination of waste products.

flavonoids A family of antioxidant chemicals found in some plants.

free radical An oxidant, an unstable atom that stabilises itself by robbing a nearby molecule, thereby creating a cascade of oxidative damage. This process is a normal part of cell workings, but in excess, is linked to ageing, heart disease, cancer and other chronic diseases.

fructo-oligo-saccharides (FOS) Indigestible, sweet-tasting, soluble fibre found in some foods that can be used as fuel by the beneficial bacteria in our intestines.

GLA (gamma linoleic acid) A fatty acid needed for healthy hormone balance, to help lower inflammation and to reduce blood clotting. Found in some plants and in evening primrose oil, it can also be made in the body from linoleic acid (found in seeds such as sunflower).

glucosinolates Chemicals naturally found in some foods, especially the brassica family (kale, (broccoli, cabbage, etc.) that help the liver's detoxification processes and act as antioxidants.

hormone Produced in a gland, this is a chemical messenger that travels via blood to sites elsewhere in the body to transmit its specific 'message' to cells.

immune system The body's complex collection of means for protecting against harmful organisms and fighting them once they are in the body.

insulin The hormone produced by the pancreas whose most important role is to help sugar (glucose) get into cells to make energy.

medium chain triglycerides (MCTs) Fats found in some foods, such as coconut, that are easily absorbed and used to make energy, and appear to help boost metabolism.

mineral Natural inorganic substance, such as iron and magnesium, found in the earth, in food and in our bodies, where they form part of the structure and function.

monounsaturated fats A type of fat, such as that found in olive oil, which has a chemical structure that makes it useful in the body and is linked to good health.

neurotransmitter A chemical messenger molecule used in the nervous system to convey messages, such as those for memory or mood, between one cell and another.

omega 3 fats A family of fats essential for healthy skin, brain, nerves, hormones and cardiovascular health, as well as lowering inflammation. Oily fish is a rich source.

omega 6 fats A family of fats (found in sunflower and pumpkin seeds, for example) that are needed in the body for healthy skin, hormones and for lowering inflammation.

oxidant A naturally occurring, unstable molecule which, if left unchecked by sufficient antioxidants, can cause damage to cells. Also known as a free radical.

pectin A type of soluble fibre found in some fruits, e.g. apples, pears and citrus fruit.

probiotic A term used to describe beneficial bacteria that we can get from quality yoghurt or in a capsule, which replenishes those we have living in our intestines.

protein Large molecules made up of specific chains of amino acids that are used in and make up the body. They are vital for structure, enzymes, neurotransmitters and transport within the body.

saturated fat (SF) Fats found in animal-derived foods that, in excess, is linked to cardiovascular disease. Coconut and palm oils also contain saturated fat.

serotonin A neurotransmitter made and used in the body, associated with good moods and sleep amongst other things.

tamari A wheat-free sauce made from the fermentation of soya beans, similar to soy sauce. Very useful for adding flavour and saltiness to savoury dishes.

tryptophan An amino acid that the body can use to make vitamin B3 and serotonin and needed for growth.

vitamin An organic micronutrient found in foods that is vital to health, normal body processes and disease prevention.

wonderfoods contacts

Natalie Savona's nutrition work
For information, visit www.nataliesavona.com

The British Society for Ecological Medicine
Promotes the study and practice of allergy, environmental and nutritional medicine.
www.bsaenm.org

Coeliac UK
The website of the charity offering advice to anyone with the condition.
www.coeliac.co.uk
Tel: 01494 437 278

Eating Disorders Association
An organisation offering information and help on all aspects of eating disorders.
www.edauk.com
Tel: 0845 634 1414 – adult helpline, 0845 634 7650 – under 18s helpline

Food Dudes
Information about the Healthy Eating Programme, and other research by the Bangor Food Research Unit at the University of Wales.
www.fooddudes.co.uk
Tel: 01248 38 3973

Green Parent
The website of a magazine whose subtitle is 'raising kids with a conscience'.
www.thegreenparent.co.uk
Tel: 01273 401012

Hyperactive children's support group
A registered charity that helps ADHD/hyperactive children and their families; Britain's leading proponent of a dietary approach to hyperactivity.
www.hacsg.org.uk

The Vegan Society
Promotes a diet and lifestyle free of animal products.
www.vegansociety.com
Tel: 01424 427393

The Vegetarian Society
The organisation responsible for promoting vegetarianism and giving advice on it.
www.vegsoc.org
Tel: 0161 925 2000

Weight Concern
A charity aiming to combat the growing prevalence of obesity, with a section on the website concerning children.
www.weightconcern.org.uk
Tel: 0207 679 6636 (no helpline service)

National Farmers' Retail & Markets Association (FARMA)
A website of the organisation that governs and promotes farmers' markets throughout the UK.
www.farmersmarkets.net
Tel: 0845 45 88 420

Henry Doubleday Research Organisation
HRDA is dedicated to researching and promoting organic gardening, farming and food.
www.hdra.org.uk
Tel: 024 7630 3517

The Soil Association
Leading organisation for the campaigning for and certification of organic food.
www.soilassociation.org
Tel: 0117 314 5000

Index